SUGAR

Damayanti Datta has worn several hats over the years: a researcher, a teacher, a communicator, a correspondent, an editor and, now, an independent writer. Starting with a PhD in history from Cambridge University, her career path has taken her towards storytelling in various fields. Over her 14 years at *India Today* magazine, she has reported from places as diverse as hospital wards, courthouses, science labs, police stations, heritage landscapes and tribal homes. She has been honoured with numerous fellowships and awards, including the first Press Council of India Award for Excellence in Investigative Journalism. *Sugar: The Silent Killer* is her maiden book on the public health disaster the ubiquitous kitchen ingredient can trigger—from diabetes to Covid-19.

SUGAR
THE SILENT KILLER

Damayanti Datta

Published by
Rupa Publications India Pvt. Ltd 2022
7/16, Ansari Road, Daryaganj
New Delhi 110002

Sales centres:
Allahabad Bengaluru Chennai
Hyderabad Jaipur Kathmandu
Kolkata Mumbai

Copyright © Damayanti Datta 2022

The views and opinions expressed in this book are the author's own and the facts are as reported by her which have been verified to the extent possible, and the publishers are not in any way liable for the same.

All rights reserved.
No part of this publication may be reproduced, transmitted, or stored in a retrieval system, in any form or by any means, electronic, mechanical, photocopying, recording or otherwise, without the prior permission of the publisher.

While every effort has been made to verify the authenticity of the information contained in this book, it is not intended as a substitute for medical consultation with a physician.
The publisher and the author are in no way liable for the use of the information contained in this book.

ISBN: 978-93-5520-300-7

First impression 2022

10 9 8 7 6 5 4 3 2 1

The moral right of the author has been asserted.

Printed in India

This book is sold subject to the condition that it shall not, by way of trade or otherwise, be lent, resold, hired out, or otherwise circulated, without the publisher's prior consent, in any form of binding or cover other than that in which it is published.

In memory of my father

Contents

Foreword	*ix*
Preface	*xi*
1. An Inheritance of Sugar	1
2. Should You Be Afraid of Sugar?	22
3. Blooms, Bees and Sugar, Please	41
4. Sweet Cravings of a Stone Age Brain	59
5. What Sugar Really Does to You	77
6. Sugar and the Slow Burn	96
7. The Great Nutrition Transition	114
8. A Virus That Loves Sugar	132
9. Eating with the Gods	147
Acknowledgements	169
Notes	171

Foreword

As evidenced by the earliest human settlements, with the evolution of human habitat, our food and eating habits too have evolved. The foods consumed have changed in form, undergoing processing, staying distant from the natural produce. The nature of physical activity has also transformed sharply with mechanization and advancement in tools and technologies. We have now crossed the cusp of eating fresh food, relying heavily on processed and preserved foods.

The tectonic shift in lifestyle coupled with eating habits has distinctly shown its effect on our health. Infectious diseases, thanks to advancements in the medical field, are minimal, while lifestyle disorders and chronic diseases have become rampant.

Sugar is one of the foremost food ingredients wreaking havoc on our health. With our obsession for sweets and the increased intake of refined sugar, metabolic and other disorders have forced us to relook at the rapidity of changing healthcare challenges.

In her book *Sugar: The Silent Killer*, Damayanti Datta has captured and discussed at length, the historical aspects of sugar extraction, the socio-cultural significance of a variety of sweets and the impact sugar has on our civilization. This is no sugar-coated tablet, but a bitter pill of truth served with a genuine concern for our well-being, warning us of the disastrous effects if we do not reform our habits and restrain our palate.

During her journalistic sojourn, interactions with people from different professions and backgrounds have helped Damayanti in aggregating a wealth of information into flowing prose of vivid description. The warning is worth heeding and I am sure this eye-opener of a book will serve handy for people of all ages to remain conscious of their diet and reclaim healthy ways of living.

Dr Devi Prasad Shetty
Renowned cardiac surgeon and Chairman of Narayana Health chain of hospitals. He was awarded the Padma Bhushan in 2012 for his contribution to the field of affordable healthcare.

Preface

This is the story of sugar. A story I have told my sister every morning over coffee in the last two years. A story I tell my friends over the phone, whenever I get the chance. A story for myself and people like me, who tuck into convenient comfort foods—full of sugar and poor carbohydrates—when a stressful day takes its toll, or raid the fridge at the dead of night because we are awake, burning the midnight oil.

This is a story for people like us, because a time comes when our bodies start sending signals and suddenly we lose the illusion that diseases and death cannot happen to us. This is, then, a story for those (like me), who wake up with new goals in life: of eating right, living clean, keeping the immune system fighting fit, the gut microbiome well-nourished, inflammation levels calm and stress at bay, so that we can compress morbidity and attain optimum health.

This is also the story of a great nation. Let's call it the 'Republic of Sugar'. If anything unites its 1.3 billion people in their diversity, it is the collective penchant for sweet taste. A civilizational obsession of an ancient land, where nature has been bountiful. For thousands of years, people have learnt to conquer bees to procure honey, tap date palms to gather golden jaggery and domesticate wild sugar cane grass to innovate crystals of sugar. Gazing up at the stars and contemplating the cosmos, they have sung their sacred hymns, celebrating the joy of sweetness.

Unfortunately, the taste of sweet is a complex phenomenon. The body needs sugar to keep ticking. Sugar coats every living cell in our body and plays a key role in every biological process. The brain can't function without sugar and rewards the body with pleasure hormones for consuming more and more of it. With sugar as our prime source of energy, sweet taste is one of the most passionate (even addictive) sensations we experience. But what happens when excess sugar becomes an acquired habit over millennia?

In 1831, a slim volume grandly titled *Pakrajeshwar*, or the Lord of the Kings of Culinary Art, was published in Calcutta (now Kolkata). It was the first printed cookbook of the country, drawing inspiration from culinary traditions that blossomed in the royal palaces of medieval Hindu and Muslim rulers. It had its share of pulaos, kebabs and dum pukhts, but overshadowing the sumptuous delights was something else—a vast and spectacular array of desserts. Baked, fried, steamed, cooked, garnished, stuffed or granulated, the sweet feast between the pages of the book expressed best what it had to say about its country: a place with a ravenous sweet tooth.

Today, the country's affinity for the 'sweet stuff' continues unabated, way above the global standard. Sweetness is not just a taste for us; it is an unconscious language of conversation, of values and beliefs that nourish our collective mind and soul. We still feed newborns sweet, creamy rice gruel as the first food. We propitiate gods and guests with sweet servings, we mark every rite of passage with sweets and we sweeten the mouth to share good news or to bribe our way out of a tight spot.

With industrialization and the fast-food revolution, 'added sugar' now hides everywhere in the food supply, making our diets increasingly unhealthy. We trade off food that is good for our health for food that tastes good. We feast on processed foods loaded with refined cereals, added sugar and sugar-sweetened drinks, but few nutrients. Nutrition habits may have gone through dramatic changes, but the human genome—the blueprint of our life that has evolved over millennia—has not had enough time to adapt to our modern eating habits.

The result is a public health disaster. Pills, patches and pricks have become the daily companions of a large number of people. They are the citizens of a country that tops the world in diseases linked to sugar (and the fat with which sugar is inextricably linked): from obesity to diabetes, heart disease to hypertension, cancers to dementia. Sugar has also ravaged them in the war between mankind and pathogens. For the new virus, SARS-CoV-2, which causes Covid-19, each step in its life cycle is paved by sugar. And it has found easy victims in people worn down by excessive sugar in their blood.

Why is there so little awareness about the destruction sugar can cause to the human body? Apart from taste, there seems to be nothing redeeming about those little white crystals. If sugar is really so bad, why is it so deeply entrenched in our food system? Shouldn't doctors, policymakers and activists rise as one to challenge sugar—

as with tobacco and alcohol? I asked a friend of mine who is a doctor: 'Why don't doctors tell us how bad sugar really is for us?' I was flummoxed by his answer: 'Because you guys never ask.'

The era of not asking questions is over. In fact, the questions are now coming from within the scientific community. In 2013, the *British Medical Journal* raised the bold question: is sugar the real culprit in the obesity epidemic? It was in response to research that highlighted the toxic, addictive and appetite-driving properties of sugar. There are scientists who are calling sugar as harmful as cocaine. Sugar, they say, needs to be taxed, just as tobacco products are. Sugar, to them, is a poison that enters our food chain in massive quantities, thanks to the food industry, and plays havoc with our health.

There are others who point to nutrition transitions (or fundamental changes in the way people eat) that damage sustainable agricultural systems and healthy eating patterns. Quick adoption of technology, high-yielding seeds, intensive farming and chemical fertilizers, for instance, have brought down the consumption of traditional coarse grains, pulses and millets—the mainstay of Indian diets for millennia as well as inexpensive sources of energy and protein for the masses. Similar changes have been seen in China and Brazil, pushing up carbohydrate consumption (which turns into sugar in the body) in a chain reaction.

Writing this book has truly been a learning experience. Without it, I may not have discovered late Dr John Yudkin, the outspoken British doctor, who sounded the alarm about the dangers of sugar in the 1970s but was ridiculed and sidelined. His hypothesis is gaining ground once again. This book has also made me dig into our ancient eating traditions and explore public health messages hidden in the 'foods of the gods'. Above all, it has inspired me to question everything I put in my mouth, cut down on sugar as much as possible and align my eating patterns with my sleep–wake rhythms. If it does the same to you, my purpose would be served.

1
An Inheritance of Sugar

It was April 2020. A sinister virus was marching outward from China. Every day was bringing unexpected news and impossible experiences. A curious report caught my eye. It seemed, while life was upending in chaos, culinary experiments were going on in my city, Calcutta, with more than a little imagination and a lot of sugar. Veteran confectioners were innovating a new type of sweet to mark the coronavirus crisis: the *corona sandesh*. With angry, red layers of icing and a crown of sugary spikes, it looked just like its namesake virus, SARS-CoV-2.

My city has a reputation for eccentricity and off-centre humour, relished and cultivated historically.[1] Sweets have been a particularly fertile field for zaniness. How else do you explain political sweets, complete with symbols and slogans, ahead of every election? Sweet surprises greet us at every outburst of popular enthusiasm. Tales of wonder creations have become a part of the city's gastronomic memory—from the discovery of the roshogolla in the nineteenth century, to the creation of *Bulganiner bishmoy* (Bulganin's wonder) in 1955 during Soviet premier Marshal Bulganin's visit to the city.[2] The corona sandesh segues neatly into this idiosyncratic world. Or does it really?

Cue the double entendre: the word 'sandesh' means 'news' in Sanskrit. In my part of India, Bengal (and Bangladesh, from which it was partitioned in 1947), sandesh is also a genre of sweets with a delicate taste and texture, suggesting glad tidings and happy promise. Gently cooked in a hundred different ways with fresh, unripened cheese, and a range of sugars, spices, fruits, nuts and flavours, the sandesh thrives on innovation. With indulgent names that sound like poetry titles, this sweet is considered the opiate of the masses in Bengal and even the emblem of Bengaliness.[3] What makes the corona sandesh an exception is the whiff of bad news around it (not to mention its prosaic name).

What's even more surprising is that the corona sandesh comes at a time when the business environment is the most precarious. The sweets business thrives on visual gluttony, aromatic seduction and over-the-counter rapport. Challenged severely by social distancing and lockdowns, customers have largely stayed away, cash flow has dwindled, artisans have fled and gallons of milk have gone down the drains (literally). Many shops have had to close down shutters. Despite some leeway from the government during the lockdowns, most shops offer a limited repertoire even now.

Why, then, are the city's prominent confectioners investing in imagination and craftsmanship in such anxious times? The answer comes from masterful thinkers of food behaviour, especially Claude Lévi-Strauss, who introduced the concept that food is more than just what we eat: for something to be 'good to eat' (*bon à manger*), it has to be first of all 'good to think' (*bon à penser*).[4] To the French anthropologist, each society's cuisine is like an unconscious language—of conversations, identities, values and beliefs—that structures their daily lives and nourishes the collective mind.

You realize that sweetness is not just pleasing to the taste but a lot more, when you speak to Rabindra Kumar Paul, the 70-something owner of Hindusthan Sweets in Calcutta, who first came up with the idea of the corona sandesh. He says he conceived the sandesh as daily bulletins of death and devastation started pouring in: 'What's better than devouring and digesting the fear of the virus?' He has also come up with poetic slogans—refashioning lines from Rabindranath Tagore—and distributes those to his customers: '*Nai, nai bhoy, hobe hobe joy, coronar hobe porajoy* (Drop all fear, victory is near, corona will be defeated).'

He is not alone. Across the world, the pandemic has unleashed a wave of creativity: people have put up original videos of activities on social media, jotted down lockdown diaries, played tennis across rooftops, helped the hungry and the homeless, and gone online to work, teach, learn, inform and entertain. Firms have come up with new ways to manage business in the wake of the disruption. And no disease has been investigated so intensely by so much combined scientific intellect as Covid-19. Psychologists call this 'meaning-making' through creative expressions in the face of an existential crisis: we turn to things that comfort us, inspire hope, and make us reflect upon who we are and what we truly value.[5]

Historically, when faced with negative emotions, uncertainty about the future or financial anxiety, people turn to food—called 'comfort foods'—to regulate their feelings. This trend has been documented after the September 11 attacks in the United States, during economic downturns and now with the Covid-19 pandemic.[6] Scholars suggest, comfort food is context dependent and differs from people to people, but they are essentially our favourite foods with a nostalgic or sentimental appeal—foods that remind us of our childhood, home, family, the good times we have had, and also generate a sense of belonging.[7]

That brings us to the question of sugar. Comfort food typically has high calorie content, a soothing taste, and a pleasant fragrance and texture. Our brain associates these sensory cues as harbingers of happiness.[8] Comfort food also promises solace, a sense of familiarity, cordiality and harmony. 'Mrs J. Haldar', a popular food columnist of *The Statesman* in the 1920s, calls sweets 'an emblem of hospitality' in every stratum of society in Bengal: 'Go to the remotest village and ask for a glass of water simply. You will have it sure, but not without sweets—be they a few pieces of sugarcandy or fondants (*batasa*).'[9]

An important trigger leading to the consumption of comfort food is when we experience loneliness, say scientists.[10] A number of studies have reported that we consume more sweet foods when we are stressed or depressed.[11] Covid-19 has proved to be particularly brutal not just for what it does to the body but also for its potential effect on the mind—isolation, loneliness, boredom and a sense of larger disconnect with the world.

In this context, the story of a new sweet, a sweet-loving city and one man's effort to deal with a deadly virus through what he knows best, becomes an intriguing (but not all that eccentric) moment in the pandemic.

The Republic of Sugar

It's a story with layers to peel back. For, the corona sandesh puts the spotlight squarely on sugar and India's ravenous appetite for it. Away from the spotlight, the reality is more complex, for sugar is not *just* sugar. There is prehistory, history, religion, culture, language, memory, economics, politics, science and diseases that make sugar, sugar. That explains why the world consumes so much of it and why India's affinity for the sweet stuff is way above any other country, if both traditional and modern sugars are counted.[12]

We also take excessive amounts of poor-quality carbohydrates (bad carbs), especially, refined cereals like white rice and white wheat, sugar-sweetened drinks and fruit juice, sweet treats and savouries, which ultimately turn into glucose, a simple sugar used by the body for energy.[13] Not surprisingly, Indians manifest an increased predilection for diseases linked to sugar (and the fat with which sugar is inextricably linked): from obesity, diabetes, heart disease and hypertension, to cancers, dementia, Covid-19 and black fungus.

The excessive consumption of sugar in India has come under severe scrutiny in the recent reports of the EAT–Lancet Commission.[14] It's a platform where the world's top scientists have debated a single question:

can the world's exploding population be fed a healthy diet within planetary boundaries?[15] By 2050, the world will be home to approximately 10 billion people, reports the World Bank. Our food systems will not be able to meet the nutritional demands of that massive population without irreversibly damaging the planet. The only way out is through collective action: transforming our eating habits, improving food production and reducing food waste.

Sugar has played a starring role in scholarly works in the West ever since the American anthropologist Sidney W. Mintz called it a massive demographic force in world history.[16] The role of sugar in the Atlantic slave trade, the Industrial Revolution as well as the fast-food revolution has been the subject of much research.[17] Hundreds of books have been written on diabetes and dietary advice. An explosion of scientific research has emerged on the shifting winds of nutrition around the world, with sugar playing a key role in it. For instance, researchers are now exploring how in the 1960s, the sugar lobby paid scientists to downplay the role of sugar in heart disease.[18]

India has had a long association with sugar—the origin of sugar cane goes back 3,500 years in our country as compared with only a thousand years in the West. Yet, there have been very few attempts to understand sugar's hold on us. Books have been written mainly on the sugar industry, and some on diabetes and low-sugar diets. This book attempts to fill the lacunae between them. It attempts to demystify the way we eat now, and the pre-eminence of refined sugar in our diet, what it does to us and what we can do to mitigate its malign influence. Weaving together history, culture and science, it seeks to analyse why we have such an intimate relation with sugar, why it holds on to us so doggedly and why we can't do without it, even when we know it can harm us in so many ways.

Is it right to focus on a single component like sugar? Human nutrition is, after all, exceedingly complex. We eat tangled combinations of nutrients as food. It's hard to pinpoint a single ingredient as the sole cause of a disease, as problems like obesity, diabetes or heart disease develop over a lifetime. Is it possible, then, to separate a single item from our dietary pattern? Is it even feasible to fathom the impact of one element in a diet? Seemingly similar foods can vary immensely in their nutrition profile. For example, the milk and sugar content of a home-made sandesh is different from that of a store-bought one. Recent research, however, shows that foods high in sugar are markers of poor diet quality. And eating patterns marked by high quantity of these are negatively associated with health.[19]

What is the way out? Instead of banishing one food ingredient from your life, examine the underpinnings of what you eat. Ask yourself who you are, where you have come from, and what is your history and your personality, to figure out how sugar influences the food decisions you take. Like the English poet William Blake, who saw the world in a grain of sand, place yourself within the collective dynamic of sugar craving in your community to understand your own instincts, impulses and yearnings. The corona sandesh has made me dig into my past to do just that. It has also provided me with the starting point to this book: the culture of collective sweet tooth I have inherited.

Memories of Comfort

My favourite poem growing up was one that conjured up visions of an unnameable sweet feast: juicy, sun-dried mango pulp (*aamshotto*), layers peeled and dropped into creamy milk, a hearty mash-up of bananas, a touch of tender sandesh and sounds of supreme relish. I loved the last line about heartbroken ants shedding tears on the empty plate. The living drama over a sugar-laden plate was, in fact, a couplet, written by Tagore as a child.[20] That a man who looked like a saint with flowing robes and beard in his photographs and whose songs and poems were on every lip, could revel in gluttony over sweets, never failed to stir my imagination.

Not just imagination, sweets made up a world of sensory experiences: visually, there was no end to their shapes and sizes—triangles, squares, oblongs, diamonds, ovals, rounds, cubes, drums, popcorns, folded, moulded and innumerable combinations of these. It was also a world of deliciousness that went beyond sweetness: complex combinations of flavours and textures from sweets made of milk products, flour and pulses fried in ghee, that could both melt and crunch in the mouth. Then there were aromas and fragrances that were pure magic: of sugar syrup on the boil, of cardamom, cloves and camphor, of fruit pulps and nuts, and the heady whiff of fresh *nolen gur*.[21]

Our lives tilted on a sweet axis, so to say. Sweets were

always stocked at home for anyone who dropped by. A social visit to relatives and friends without sweets was considered rude. Endless supplies of home-made sticky-crunchy orbs of deliciousness—*moa* and *naru*, made of jaggery, puffed or flattened rice, sesame or coconuts—were our mainstay on happy afternoons over storybooks. The sandesh inevitably accompanied us to school in our lunch box every day. And we waited eagerly for the hawker, who came with a straw basket on his head, full of the crescent-shaped, coconut *chandrapuli sandesh* and the moist balls of sweet, popped rice—*Jaynagarer moa*.

Every rite of passage had to have sweets. *Payesh (payaas)*—made of rice, milk and sugar—was a must-have at the first rice-eating ceremony of infants and also at birthdays. Wedding trousseaus included decorated trays of assorted sweets. In my family, a tin full of intricately carved stone *chhach* (mould) of flowers, fishes, butterflies and mythical creatures was brought out at every family wedding. Brushed with ghee, the moulds were used to make *khirer chhacher sandesh,* a speciality of the women of Sylhet (in present-day Bangladesh). A new bride was welcomed with a touch of honey on her mouth and ears so that words, said and heard, would be sweet. Funeral tributes meant garlands of rajanigandha flowers on the photograph of the deceased, lighting of incense sticks and offerings of sandesh.

The insatiable appetite for sweets transgressed the boundaries between the sacred and the profane. While temples prepared payesh for the gods, devotees sought blessings with flowers and sweets (*peda*) stuffed in straw baskets. During Durga Puja, heaps of sweets did the rounds and ended with women touching the mouth of the Devi with sandesh to bid her a symbolic goodbye. The distribution of unlimited sweets followed the immersion of the idol in the Ganges, as people embraced, greeted and saluted each other with cries of '*Shubho Bijoya*' (Happy Bijoya) to celebrate the triumph of good over evil. Like other women, my mother prepared special sweetmeats at home during these festivities. One such sweet to die for was *ichar mura*. Made of coconut, caramelized milk, spices and ghee on slow fire, it was named for its resemblance to prawn heads.

On Bhai Phonta, sisters wished for the longevity of their brothers with a dot of sandalwood paste on their foreheads and platters of sweets. On Jamai Sasthi, mothers-in-law felicitated their sons-in-law with a sumptuous luncheon and, of course, sweet treats. On Poush Parbon, a traditional harvest festival to commemorate the winter solstice, families gathered to feast on sweets made of grated coconut and newly harvested honey-gold nolen gur: *malpoa, patishapta, pithe* and payesh. Every family brought out its terracotta pithe moulds from the pantry at this time, a tradition linking us across centuries to the harvest festivals narrated in the medieval verses of the *Mangal Kavya*[22].

More broadly, the word *mishti* (sweet) stood for a universe of things that looked, felt or smelt good—be it fragrance, colour, nature, music, voice, disposition, behaviour, affection and even anger in romance. Girls were routinely named 'Mishti' or 'Mishtu'. '*Mishti meye*' was a way to describe a pretty girl. Language and literature reflected the importance of sweets in our lives.

Phrases and idioms like '*mukh mishti*' (which ranged in meaning from sweet words to sharing one's happiness by treating others to sweets), '*michhrir chhuri*' (a honeyed dagger, for people cloaking evil intentions with sweet words) or '*mone jilipir pyanch*' (to be as convoluted as the rings of the syrupy *jilipi*), were part of everyday parlance. An entertaining proverb was, '*Notun notun khoier moa kachar machar kore*' (moa of newly made popped rice makes a lot of noise), implying upstarts who show off new wealth.

The most popular children's magazines of the day, where we vied to get our stories and sketches published, were called *Sandesh* and *Mouchak*, both names of sweets.[23] Our favourite movie was Satyajit Ray's *Goopy Gyne Bagha Byne*, where hundreds of clay pots heaped with sweets rained down magically from the sky on a battlefield—the climax heralding peace. I avidly read the exploits of the detective duo Jayanta-Manik in mystery books written by Hemendra Kumar Roy, laughing uproariously at the stupidities of the unfit police officer who accompanied them and dug into sweets whenever he could. My favourite book was Abanindranath Tagore's fairy tale, *Khirer Putul*, where a clever monkey used the sly subterfuge of a doll made of *kheer* (milk slow-cooked until thick) to help a neglected queen regain her glory.

A story I heard growing up about my city's craze for sweets was also my father's favourite: it was about a 'sweet revolt' in Calcutta, when sweets made of milk were banned by the Gandhian chief minister, Prafulla Chandra Sen, in August 1965, under the West Bengal Channa Sweets Control Order. With mounting public rage, Sen had even delivered a speech on All India Radio justifying the legislation in view of a tough economic environment. Both the order and his speech incensed people so much that he was challenged in the Calcutta High Court, with the judges coming down heavily on him. Within a year, he and his party lost in the assembly elections.[24] All for banning milk sweets? Maybe, maybe not, but the banning of milk sweets certainly tipped public opinion against him.

Delights of a Godforsaken Land

For millennia before I was born, an accident of geography and history had created a people with a bad case of sweet tooth. They lived in isolation in a marshy land surrounded by dense forests, disconnected hill systems and a myriad of waterways, including some of the largest rivers in South Asia: the Ganges, the Brahmaputra and the Meghna. An inaccessible eastern frontier to the North Indian plains since time immemorial, it was linked to the rest of the Indian subcontinent with only three hazardous passes—Teliagarhi, Tirhut and Jharkhand—before the advent of the railways in the nineteenth century.[25]

The region was peripheral not just in location, but also as a discursive construct. It was unknown to the composers of the Rig Veda. Later, Vedic texts scorned it as a land of barbarians, where rites and cults of animism, totem and magic were practised. Agni, the God of Fire, refused to cross the frontier.[26] In Patanjali's *Mahabhashya* (second century BCE), it was excluded from the land of the Aryans, or what was known as Aryavarta. This exclusion ensured that caste system remained relatively flexible within this territory. Brahmins here ate fish and meat, which was frowned upon elsewhere, and wrote texts justifying their eating habits.[27]

The vantage point gave rise to a distinctive regional identity.[28] In the Mahabharata war, the region allied with the anti-heroes, the Kauravas. The Nastika school of philosophy, which like Buddhism, Jainism and Ajivika rejects the authority of the Vedas, flourished.[29] Tantric mysticism, which spurns caste and patriarchy, exerted a strong hold, democratizing society, and giving right of worship to women and people down the class and caste ladder. Folk pantheons and the tradition of goddess worship found new clout and legitimacy. Challenging the mainstream was so endemic here that under the Mughals, the region even came to be known as the 'home of revolts'.[30]

Identity played out at the intersection of folkways and food ways. Distinctive culinary habits based on the availability of local ingredients as well as new cultural and gastronomic influences, created a cuisine that was pluralistic yet their own. Rice grew abundantly in the fertile floodplains. The medieval text, *Shunya Purana*, mentions 50 different varieties of rice grown in this region. Rice—boiled, puffed, flattened or parched—was their abiding staple. And they loved fish, a nod to pre-Aryan linkages in a riverine landscape.[31] The first Bengali text, the *Charyapada*, composed between tenth and twelfth century CE, described fishing and hunting, apart from a range of food crops, vegetables and fruits. *Matsya* (fish), *mamsa* (meat) and *mudra* (parched grains) were also among the five Ms enjoined by Tantra.[32]

People spent an enormous amount of time, energy—and, yes, emotion—on food and cooking: from procuring, selecting, preparing, serving and eating, to thinking and talking about it. There was much play between distinctive flavours, mouthfeel and a procession of tastes in a total meal, from bitter to sweet.[33] Text after text depicted the eating culture of the region. A verse from *Prakrita Paingala,* a thirteenth-century text from Bengal, mentioned the idea of a fulfilled man: 'Fortunate is the man whose wife serves him on a banana leaf hot rice with ghee, *mourala* fish, fried leaf of jute plant, and hot milk.'[34]

This culinary imagination was not just a matter of preference. It was resistance to the colonization of taste, too.[35] It allowed the region to break taboos and set new styles in motion with every new influence: political, religious or entrepreneurial. For instance, the injunctions of the *Smriti* writers on cooked fish and meat were recommended by the eleventh-century physician and commentator of Ayurveda, Chakrapanidatta.[36] The most visible example of their cosmopolitan culinary identity was, perhaps, of using *chhana* (or unripened cheese) as a medium for sweets after the arrival of the Portuguese in the sixteenth century. The Vedic taboo on the deliberate curdling of milk was broken only here. Chhana became the defining element of Bengali dessert ever since.

Chhana was the last ingredient to be added to the perfect storm of sweet tastes and flavours that marked the region since ancient times. It was the original seat of the high-quality sugar cane Paundra or Paundraka mentioned in the second century BCE medical text *Charaka Samhita.*

From sugar cane came the name Paundra Vardhana, the ancient kingdom of northern Bengal, with poets singing paeans to the beauty of sugar cane fields.[37] The art of making sugar cane juice and sugar was applied to the *madhuka* flower (*mahua*) and date palm (*khejur*) as well.

It was in the fitness of things that a land famous for the cultivation of sugar cane had its ancient name, Gauda, after a key sugar cane product: *gur* or molasses. The seventh-century Tang emperor of China, Tai-Hung, sent emissaries to learn the art and craft of sugar making from India (*Lyu*) and especially Bengal (*Mo-Ki-To*).[38] Medieval literature testified to the region's long-standing fascination for all things sweet. One felt like a king, went a verse in *Prakrita Paingala*, with enough clarified butter (*ghitta*) to prepare 20 cakes of fried sweets (*pistaka*).[39] Up to the eighteenth century, sugar was a key item of flourishing trade in Bengal with coastal Africa, the Persian Gulf, Southeast Asia, Tibet and China.[40]

It was, however, an aromatic variety of molasses from the sap of silver date palm (*Phoenix sylvestris*) that made their sweets truly different. Sourcing palm sap for making wine or toddy was widely practised across the world since ancient times, but it harmed the trees. What developed in this region was an unusual skill: tapping the tree, without harming it, for jaggery—variously called, *khejur gur*, nolen gur, *jhola gur* or *patali gur*.[41] Perfected over centuries, a specialized profession of tree tappers emerged, who knew when to climb the trees in winter, how to make the right incisions and where to tie clay pots to collect the sap overnight. They also knew how long to churn the sap in iron cauldrons, until it gave off the right heady aroma and turned into a viscous golden syrup.

Sweets also marked the flexibility of the culture to changing times and tastes: Islamic, Christianity and Jewish, to name a few. Cookbooks tell this unusual story. The first printed cookbook in an Indian language was written in Bangla in 1831. Grandly titled *Pakrajeshwar,* or the Lord of the Kings of Culinary Art, it claimed to draw inspiration from culinary traditions that blossomed in the royal palaces of King Vikramasena of sixteenth-century Ujjain, fifth Mughal emperor Shah Jahan and Alivardi Khan, the nawab of Bengal (1740–56). It listed 16 types of sweets—*ladduka* and *gulab jamun* to *jilipi*—indicating a syncretic eating tradition, where food did not divide, rather accommodated many worlds.[42]

The most popular cookbook in the late nineteenth century, *Pak-Pranali,* written by one Bipradas Mukhopadhyay, similarly depicted a wide range of age-old and new sweets.[43] The list of ingredients stretched over two pages, with 38 different varieties of milk products and 18 types of sugar. Of the recipes, the book mentioned 17 types of sweets cooked with ghee; 20 types made with *besan, suji, maida,* rice powder or hung *dahi* (curd); 23 layered sweets like *khaja* and *gaja*; 26 types of *barfi* and *mohanbhog*; 13 types of fruit *morabba*; 23 types of sandesh; 45 types of payesh and pishtak; 45 types of sweet beverages; and 22 types of miscellaneous sweets.

At the heart of the craze for sweets lay artisanal curiosity, creativity and a sense of community. For the sweet-making communities of *moira* and *modak,* it meant success. For centuries, sweet making was a traditional industry in this region. With the piety advocated by Sri Chaitanya's Bhakti movement in the sixteenth century, the abundance of milk-based sweets (the favourite food of Lord Krishna and Lord Vishnu) that were taken and shared by Sri Chaitanya among his followers across caste, class, community and gender, brought the sweet-makers prestige and esteem.

New sacred sites, patronage networks, pilgrim spots and associated village fairs sprung up, widening their opportunities for movement and trade. For instance, the Malla kings of Bishnupur, who ruled over a vast stretch in of south-western Bengal, were known for their patronage of terracotta architecture, silk weaving, the Bishnupur *gharana* of classical music and their influence on sweets.[44] When the royals embraced Vaishnavism in the sixteenth century, they brought in milkmen and confectioners from other areas and settled them around the new Vishnu temples they built in order to create new sweets for worship and offerings.[45]

An unmistakable enthusiasm over new gastronomic possibilities marked the history of the region from then on. 'Entire streets could be seen wholly occupied by skilled sweetmeat-makers who proved their skill by offering wonderful sweet-scented dainties of all kinds, which would stimulate the most jaded appetite to gluttony,' wrote Sebastian Manrique, the seventeenth-century Portuguese missionary and traveller.'[46] The landed elite of Bengal patronized local confectioners. Distinctive sweets originated in different areas, dotting the region with unique sweets, each with its own story and individuality: the *jalbhora talsansh sandesh*, shaped like a palm kernel and filled with nolen gur, under the zamindars of Telinipara; the granular *sitabhog* and *mihidana* under the Maharaja of Bardhaman; the *monohara* in Janai and so on.[47]

Calcutta, the erstwhile capital of the British Empire, attracted creative confectioners. One Paran Chandra Nag created the sandesh and sold it in his shop in 1826. His son Bhim Chandra Nag added to his father's repertoire and built up a formidable reputation. The momentum was propelled by a group of talented and enterprising confectioners. The business was driven by innovation and patronage of preferred clientele: Bhim Chandra, for instance, created *ledikeni*, a fried reddish-brown sweet ball, for the Vicereine Lady Charlotte Canning; one Nobin Chandra Das whipped up the delectable *abaar khabo* for the dowager Maharani Swarnamoyee of Kasimbazar. Nobin Chandra's signature sweet, roshogolla, became a marker of Bengali gastronomic identity.[48]

For the people of Calcutta, the new sweets became a feel-good factor. For some, they also served as a means to navigate through trust, distrust and family ties. Maharani Swarnamoyee, who raised the income of her estate from ₹16 lakh in 1801 to ₹30 lakh in 1897 through efficient management and shrewd diplomacy, used to send the *monoranjan sandesh* (priced at ₹12 a kilogram, the same as a Dhakai saree) to her allies as well as her foes. That was also her way to keep the volatile senior (widowed) women of the family in good humour.[49]

Many young, talented people were drawn to the art of sweet making, even if they did not belong to the caste of confectioners and had no family tradition of making sweets. One such was Nobin Chandra Das, who came from a family of sugar merchants and was shunned by his relatives for following his dream of becoming a sweet maker. Another was Ashutosh Sen, who opened a small shop in Shyam Bazaar in 1885. For 40 years, his shop did not have a name. A group of writers and poets of the city, including Sarat Chandra Chattopadhyay, Tarashankar Bandopadhyay and Banaphool (the pseudonym of Balaichand Mukhopadhyay), who gathered at his shop every evening, named it after him, Sen Mahasay or Sir Sen.[50]

In this creative assortment, there were also confectioners and sweets from outside the region: for instance, Ganguram Chaurasia, a skilled halwai from Varanasi, Uttar Pradesh, who set up the first shop to sell North Indian and Marwari sweets in 1885; Federico Peliti, an Italian who worked as the purveyor of cakes at the viceregal house since 1868, and opened the first upmarket continental restaurant and confectionery in 1881. In the twentieth century, there were four Swiss and Italian confectioneries which became institutions: Flurys, Trincas, Firpo's and Ferrazzini.[51] The Jewish Nahoum & Sons and Portuguese MX D'Gama were famous as patisseries. By this time, the English fetish for sweetened tea had spread, from railway stations to fancy tea rooms.

The one thing that went unnoticed in the ensuing culinary excitement was sugar itself. Mill-made, nutritionally inferior white sugar started appearing from the late-nineteenth century, aided by protective tariff. Despite protests, bonfires and boycott of sugar and other British-manufactured products during the Swadeshi movement of 1905, the march of the cheaper refined sugar could not be stopped. In 1907, Sir Richard Havelock Charles, a British physician stationed in India, made the alarming observation that type 2 diabetes was increasing rapidly among the wealthy Bengalis living in Calcutta, whereas it was still rare among the poor Punjabis. He linked this with an increasing intake of sugar.[52] The famous sweet tooth of the region was going out of control. Swami Vivekananda, the thoroughly modern saint with a prescient eye, wrote in his unforgiving prose:

> Formerly, our village zamindars…would think nothing of walking twenty or thirty miles, and would eat twice—twenty Koi fish bones and all—and they lived to a hundred years. Now their sons and grandsons…put on airs, wear spectacles, eat the sweets from the bazaars, hire a carriage to go from one street to another, and then complain of diabetes—and their life is cut short, this is the result of their being civilized.[53]

Has the culture of obsession with sweets given Bengal the highest rates of diabetes in India? Not really. The southern states of Tamil Nadu and Kerala top the charts, along with Delhi, followed by Punjab, Goa and Karnataka.[54] Experts have tried to explain the reasons at work, but not very convincingly. To some, Kerala has the highest percentage of elderly in the country and diabetes is typically a disease of age (although this is changing). What about Sikkim, then? It has very high prevalence of diabetes but negligible ageing population.

To others, the standard of living in Kerala has gone through rapid transition in recent years, thanks to the influx of money from the Malayali diaspora.[55] Diabetes, however, is no longer a disease of affluence. It is now a serious concern in poverty-stricken rural households, too. What about diet, then? Bengal is as fanatic about sweets as it is about fish. Research is not definitive, but some studies do show eating a lot of fatty fish, with high concentrations of omega-3 fatty acids helps reduce the risk of type 2 diabetes. Yet, this does not solve the diabetes puzzle. Kerala, like West Bengal, has the highest per capita fish consumption in India.[56]

The bottom line is, sugar is complicated. Just as complicated as we are. Our food environment, our love for new foods and fads, how we cook, from whom we buy our foods, when we eat, and how we live, work and think, everything can impact the story of sugar. The next few chapters will explore the many shades of sugar in our lives: the good, the bad and the scary.

2

Should You Be Afraid of Sugar?

Fifty years ago, a book came out. It could have changed the world. Instead, it was relegated to the trash: the author was severely criticized, even persecuted, and his message was drowned out by a chorus of deriding voices. Just because he dared to ask: why do people eat so much sugar? Why do they know so little about its dangers? He had conducted experiments on animals and people for 25 years and come to the conclusion that a lot of sugar in the diet leads to high levels of fat and insulin in the blood—now deemed as risk factors for heart disease and diabetes. The book in question was *Pure, White and Deadly: How Sugar Is Killing Us and What We Can Do to Stop It,* written by Dr John Yudkin in 1972. Even a few years ago, it was lying idle on dusty library shelves like wasted ammunition.

What made Dr Yudkin write the book was the realization that sugar was almost a black box: there were scores of books on the cultivation of sugar cane and sugar beet, and technical books and trade manuals on sugar refining and manufacture of sugar-containing foods and drinks. There were also books on the deplorable slave trade of sugar between Europe, West Africa and the Caribbean. Dr Yudkin wanted to tell the story of sugar as a food and what it does to our health. He wanted people to understand the ways in which our health gets affected under two extreme circumstances: when we take no sugar at all, and also when we take large amounts of it.

It was a time marked by an array of research on the health effects of bread, eggs, meat, breakfast cereals and vegetables in our diet. Although sugar constituted about 17 per cent of the average western diet, there were no guidelines on how much was too much. What the sugar industry consistently recommended as 'moderate' quantity of sugar in diet was 10–30 per cent of total calories—this went against his own findings. What finally triggered him to write the book was a question he was asked often: why don't we hear very much about the dangers of sugar, while we are constantly being told we have too much fat in our diet, and not enough fibre?[1]

Dr Yudkin was born in 1910 to parents who had fled anti-Jewish violence of the Russian pogroms of 1905 to settle down in London. He did his matriculation at Christ's College, Cambridge University, as a scholar, and graduated in biochemistry in 1931, at the age of 20. On completing his medical studies in 1938, he was appointed director of Medical Studies at Christ's. In 1945, the premier medical journal, *Nature*, announced his appointment to the chair of physiology at King's College, University of London.[2]

Nutrition and public health were his passion. In 1942, he wrote an article in *The Times*, London, pointing out the absence of a single body or council responsible for formulating a uniform plan of nutrition in the United Kingdom (UK). The need of the hour was a nutrition council to correct the oversight of food policy, he highlighted. Over the next several years, he persuaded his college and the University of London to establish a BSc degree in nutrition—the first such degree in any European university—in 1953. His Chair was converted into a professorship of nutrition.

What drove Dr Yudkin throughout his life was making science available to the public. The series of books he wrote between 1958 and 1990 occupies a unique place as some of the first popular science books to shape public perception on the way people ate. He consistently alerted scientists and the media to the dangers of indiscriminate consumption of certain foods and made quality nutrition research accessible. One such effort was his 1972 book on sugar, but Dr Yudkin paid a heavy price for it. With prominent scientists joining hands with the food industry to destroy his reputation, his career suffered. By the time he died, in 1995, he was a disillusioned man—unrecognized, unrecompensed and unatoned.

The Sugar Tick-Tock

Your body is a master of time. Each tiny cell in your body goes *tick-tock* every passing second. Each organ chimes at its own pace. The master clock inside your brain goes gong by the rotation of the earth. Sunlight is the key that winds them up. Together they make possible the synchronized rhythm that is your body in harmony: your temperature, blood pressure and heart rate drop at night and surge in the morning, when your feet hit the ground; at night, the body goes in for regeneration, while at daybreak, your metabolism (all the chemical reactions in your cells that change food into energy) is switched on. You are at your most alert mid-morning, have top coordination in the early afternoon and peak muscle strength late afternoon; even your immune system is timed by your inner clocks. A masterpiece of evolution, you mess with it at your peril. That's exactly what sugar does.

Let's put first things first: your body needs sugar (glucose) to keep ticking. Of the three macronutrients in your diet—carbohydrate, protein and fat—carbs are broken down into sugar and absorbed into the bloodstream. What exactly are carbohydrates? They are molecules made of various combinations of carbon, hydrogen and oxygen, which your body is capable of breaking down for energy. In fact, they are the preferred source of primary energy for all the cells in our body. It's an umbrella term for all the different types of sugars: simple sugars (glucose, fructose and galactose), carbs with complex chemical structures (say, starch) and fibre.

Your body breaks down all sugars in the same way, but simple carbs are fast-digesting and quickly boost blood sugar levels. Too many simple carbs can contribute to weight gain and also increase your risk of diabetes, heart disease and high cholesterol. Complex carbs take a bit longer, keep you feeling full for longer and give you more than just the sugar. Starches in whole grains, for instance, have vitamins, minerals and more protein. Fibres act as a gel, make the journey of digested food through your intestines slow, keep you from feeling hungry longer and help your bowel movements. Fibre is also the chief fuel for the friendly microbes in your gut.

Glucose is the major source of energy for your body. Your brain can't do without it and laps up half of all the sugar energy in your body. Your brain's capacity to think, remember and learn is closely linked to how much sugar it is getting. The brain also uses up more glucose during challenging mental tasks. Without enough sugar, the brain's chemical messengers (neurotransmitters) are not produced and communication between brain cells breaks down. Your behaviour, learning and memory become erratic too. The best sugars for the brain are complex carbs.

The 37.2 trillion cells of our bodies rely on sugar to hum and sing with energy. It's not as simple as that, though: your energy needs keep changing and your cells have to adapt to that dynamic environment. Glucose is in short supply when, for instance, you are between meals, at night when you are not eating, when you are simply resting, when you are on a low-carb diet or when you are exercising. The body then gets sugar from other sources: from stored sugar (glycogen) in muscles and liver. When this is used up, muscle protein is broken down to create glucose in the liver. Fat is broken down by the liver to produce a fuel source called ketones.

Your body, however, is wary of sugar. It knows that too much of a good thing can spoil the best-laid biological plans. Just as you protect your worldly assets with locks and keys, your body safeguards your cells against excess sugar with a key. That key is the hormone insulin, produced by the pancreas in your gut. This is how it works: when you eat, sugar enters your bloodstream, but it can't get into your cells on its own. Only when the key (insulin) opens the doors can your cells burn up the sugar as energy, for you to laugh, cry, move and think. Insulin, therefore, brings down the amount of sugar in your blood.

What happens if your cells refuse to obey the diktats of insulin? You would be insulin-resistant. Your physician may say you have metabolic syndrome—a medical condition marked by high blood pressure, high blood sugar levels, abnormal cholesterol levels and too much abdominal fat. In fact, the first symptom your doctor would look for is an expanding waistline. There is a good chance that you have metabolic syndrome if you are overweight. And you are more likely to have a heart attack or develop diabetes (or both) if you have metabolic syndrome.

What happens when sugar levels go up in your blood? Your brain detects this surge through its spies and reporters across the body. It uses the nerve system to tell your pancreas to produce insulin (imagine a high-powered telephone call from the prime minister to get things moving). Small isles of cells in the pancreas produces two hormones—insulin and glucagon—that work in tandem to ensure blood sugar levels remain within set limits and the body is able to function well. While insulin's job is to lower blood sugar levels if needed, glucagon's role is to raise blood sugar levels if they dip too low.

Your body has to work harder when you overeat foods that raise your blood sugar. Insulin tries to remove sugar as much as possible. If you continue with perilous eating habits, your pancreas responds by pumping out more and more insulin. Having elevated insulin levels persistently has harmful effects of its own, heart disease, for one. Another result is high blood pressure, higher triglyceride (a type of fat that is an important measure of your heart health) levels and lower levels of 'good cholesterol' or HDL (high-density lipoprotein). All these worsen insulin resistance further, giving you metabolic syndrome.

Slowly and progressively over time, as sugar rises in your blood, it damages the proteins, fats and even the blueprint of your body (the DNA) that make up your cells. Some excess sugar turns to fat (your body is remarkably good at storing excess sugar in the form of fat). Sugar appears in your urine. Your body fights back, produces more insulin and tries to mop up more. Eventually, your pancreas can no longer keep up with the demand and exhaustion sets in. Your blood sugar then spirals out of control, leading to diabetes.

Today, as diabetes affects nearly one in every 10 individuals worldwide, modern science is adding its own discoveries: the common type 2 diabetes (when the body can't use insulin properly) and the rarer type 1 diabetes (when the body cannot make insulin). Scientists now know what makes sugar particularly scary: the chain of damaging events it can set off. As blood turns syrupy, it sucks water out of the tissues, leading to a feeling of thirst all the time. The kidneys go into an overdrive filtering out sugar, driving you to the washroom on and off. As sugar levels rise further and insulin fails to move sugar out of the bloodstream, cells start to starve—the reason why people with diabetes suddenly start losing weight. Uncontrolled, nerves start dying in the legs (the farthest from the heart) from poor circulation, leading to wounds and amputations. The viscous blood rips holes in the delicate capillaries of the kidneys as they try to squeeze the sugar out—one of the reasons why people with diabetes often end up on dialysis. The havoc it creates on blood vessels in the heart and brain leads to stroke and heart attack. A century ago, diabetes was a death sentence. Today, one simply needs insulin injections to stay alive and kicking.

The discovery of insulin in 1921 has transformed diabetes into a chronic disease. Although it allows one to live a long and productive life, unfortunately, there is no cure for this disease. If left unmonitored, it can bring a universe of complications that can even be fatal: from premature ageing, blindness, amputations, kidney failure, elevated cholesterol, skin conditions, hypertension, blood vessel damage and heart attacks to strokes. It turns out that extremely sweet or fatty foods captivate the brain in much the same way that cocaine and gambling do. Can one become a sugar addict? As scientists debate amongst themselves and until a reasonable verdict is arrived at, it's best to steer clear of sugar.

What happens to the concert of tick-tocks inside you? Excessive food consumption, particularly foods that are high in sugar and carbohydrates, dampens your body clock and imperils your health. High sugar in your blood appears to gum up the clockwork. Scientists have noted rundown clocks everywhere in people who are overweight and obese: in the heart, kidney, liver and blood vessels. New research shows how the inner layers of blood vessels get inflamed and sticky, where cells pile up.[3] The journey of blood through the clogged up, tortuous passageways sets you on a downhill course filled with health hazards.

Quite an Extraordinary Substance

'Life is difficult for people who, like myself, want to avoid sugar,' writes Dr Yudkin in his book. A slim book of 21 short chapters, *Pure, White and Deadly* deals with questions on sugar that everyone wants to know, but are rarely asked or addressed. With stunning simplicity, the author blends his life as a citizen, his perspectives as a physician and his research acumen as a scientist. The questions he raises, and his way of raising them, are as interesting as his book's prime character: sugar. His answers open new windows of curiosity on the mysterious interaction between a common food staple and the human body. And the prescriptions he provides, based on his research, are sadly relevant even 50 years later.

Is anything different about sugar? Dr Yudkin asks. He admits that while sugar has always been a constant presence in our lives, it really is quite extraordinary. It is exceptional in the way it is produced, what can be made out of it and its effects on the body. It is unique among carbs. Large amounts of carbs have been part of the human diet ever since cooking began, yet, as Dr Yudkin writes, 'It did not seem to occur to anyone that it made any difference whether this carbohydrate consisted almost entirely of starch in wheat or rice or maize, or whether the starch was gradually becoming replaced by increasing amounts of sugar.'

Why is it that the sugar industry reveals so little about the (ill) effects of sugar? Other industries which produce foods like meat and dairy have spent a great deal of money over the years to carry out or support nutritional studies on their products, even though these foods form a smaller proportion of the modern diet than sugar does. Dr Yudkin writes, 'The sugar people seem quite content to spend their money on advertising and public relations, making claims about quick energy and...simply rejecting suggestions that sugar is really harmful...to health in general.'

Sugar is no more just what you buy for cooking at home. An increasing proportion of sugar is bought as food. Industrial sugar goes to the factory and comes to us in the form of confectionery and fancily packaged convenience foods. What Dr Yudkin calls 'industrial sugar' is added sugar in today's parlance and it remains concealed insidiously in our food chain—not just for its sweet taste, but also to add shelf-life, texture, body, colour and flavour to our food. As Dr Yudkin points out: 'When you come to think of it, almost all of the tempting foods that are taken to satisfy appetite rather than hunger contain carbohydrate that is either sugar or starch. These carbohydrate-rich foods have another characteristic; they are all artificial foods that do not exist in nature.'

Here's an exercise he recommends: take a walk around a supermarket and make a list of foods with sugar among their ingredients. Leaving aside obvious items like cakes, biscuits, desserts and soft drinks, you will find sugar in almost everything: from breakfast food, pasta and pickle to soup. And in many of these, the amount of sugar is surprisingly high. You can get a fair idea by seeing where the sugar ranks in the list of ingredients. If it is first in the list, the food will contain more sugar than any other ingredients: 'The manufacturer seems to have found, or at any rate convinced himself that people like sugar with everything, and more and more of it.'

Unexpected sources of sugar are dips, sauces and spreads. Take peanut butter, for instance. Peanuts contain very little sugar; in fact, it helps decrease weight, improve blood sugar and regulate blood fats. You would expect peanut butter to have some of these properties. Unfortunately, most ready-made peanut butters are packed with added sugar. Consider tomatoes: the amount of naturally occurring sugar in tomatoes is minimal in a serving, but tomato sauce and ketchup are loaded with sugar. One tablespoon of one of the most popular brands in India contains more than one teaspoon of sugar (one teaspoon of sugar equals 4 grams, and it contains 5 grams, according to fitbit.com nutrition tracker). Now that's a lot of sugar, considering most people use closer to 2–4 tablespoons of ketchup every time.

Dr Yudkin posits two propositions, which according to him 'no one can refute': first, physiologically, you don't need to consume sugar. He writes, 'All human nutritional needs can be met in full without having to take a single spoon of white or brown or raw sugar, on its own or in any food or drink.' Our foods from natural sources contain components that can provide fuel for the body's workings. They also contain some nutrients in the way of protein, minerals and vitamins or a mixture. A cabbage gives you vitamins A and C and calcium, amongst other essentials. A piece of meat provides protein, fat, several B vitamins, iron and many other nutrients. An average person would have quite a sizeable reserve of fuel stored in their tissues from such food, and don't need to consume sugar. Sugar contains energy, and that is all.

He raises a singular question: why do we consume a dietary component (carbs) in its isolated state (sugar)? Do we take any other dietary component—say, pure protein or pure vitamin B12—and make it a part of our diet? Yet, vast areas of land worldwide are planted with sugar cane or sugar beet, instead of crops that we can eat more or less whole. The juice is then extracted, cleaned, filtered, refined and purified until we get something that is 'virtually 100 per cent sugar'. What virtue does that represent? Isn't it like cultivating pine trees instead of cabbages, and then extracting the vitamin C and eating it instead of eating cabbage? You can now claim that you have consumed absolutely pure vitamin C. The cabbage anyway would have given you other nutritional benefits apart from vitamin C, he points out.

Dr Yudkin also sounds out a warning: if only a small fraction of what is known about the effects of sugar were seen in anything else, it would be banned. Sugar can act locally on tissues in the mouth or stomach, before it is absorbed—dental disease being a manifestation. Sugar can act after it has been digested and absorbed into the blood stream. Sugar can act by changing the numbers and proportions of the trillions of different microbes that line the intestines. And its action on the intricately interrelated system of hormones and on the liver shows sugar is not just any ordinary kind of food.

The common sugar you eat is sucrose. This type of sugar hides in far too many foods, ranging from table sugar, chocolates, cakes and cookies to fast foods, soft ice creams and ready-to-drink coffee. Sucrose breaks down into glucose and fructose before being absorbed into the blood. This digestion is usually quite complete except when very large amounts are consumed when blood is repeatedly flooded with high levels of glucose and fructose, Dr Yudkin explains: '(R)efining (sugar) deceives the tongue and the appetite, and leads to over-consumption.' Partly because it is rapidly digested and partly because people so often take sugar in food and drink between meals, when there is little else in the stomach to delay absorption, thus leading to obesity and heart disease.

Fifty years later, Dr Yudkin's repeated imploration on the effect of sugar that 'future research must pursue', is finally coming true. The recognition of the special properties of fructose (whether as part of sucrose or its cheap alternative, high-fructose corn syrup [HFCS]) that over a long period of time can damage body tissues, are under intense scrutiny. Excessive consumption of sugar is being linked to a range of adverse health outcomes. We are being told, consumption of added sugar doubles fat production; sugar impacts hunger-suppressing hormones; high-sugar diet damages the gut; children who consume too much sugar are at greater risk of becoming obese, hyperactive and cognitively impaired as adults; a diet rich in fat and sugar is linked to inflammation. Sugar is addictive, and sugar overload may be a recipe for long-term problems.

Scientist versus Scientist

The era of watching diets began in the western world from the 1950s, in response to an impending public health catastrophe: heart disease. Fat took centre stage after US President Franklin D. Roosevelt died of a sudden stroke and heart failure. A series of landmark studies came up with dietary risk factors: it was observed that those who developed atherosclerosis (hardening and narrowing of arteries) had elevated levels of 'bad' LDL (low-density lipoprotein) cholesterol and low levels of 'good' HDL cholesterol. Heightened fears of heart disease fuelled a search for the dietary components responsible for the dramatic rise in diet-related diseases and death.

Nutritionists split into two polar groups: one group, led by American physiologist Dr Ancel Keys, deemed fat to be responsible for that. So influential was his theory that *Time* magazine put him on its cover in January 1961. The data acquired by him, however, was ambiguous and flawed, but the debate grabbed public imagination and influenced policymakers. The other group concurred with the views of Dr Yudkin, that carbohydrates, primarily refined sugar, was the villain. It was an all-out war: Dr Keys secured positions for himself and his allies on the boards of the most influential bodies in American healthcare.

From his vantage point, Dr Keys rubbished Dr Yudkin's work as 'a mountain of nonsense', accusing him of using very high amounts of sugar in his lab experiments to manipulate the results and even of taking undue benefits from the meat and dairy industries.[4] Dr Yudkin wrote in his book that many people have criticized him and his work, and Dr Keys was one amongst them. In the decades that saw an intense battle play out between the two groups, Dr Keys won the day and Dr Yudkin's prophecy remained unheeded—until now.

From the 1970s, dietary guidelines started cutting down on fat of all sorts. That did not stop heart disease from spiralling out of control or an obesity crisis flaring up from the 1980s. The food industry responded by going low fat but compensated for taste by loading up on added sugars and artificial sweeteners. Between 1962 and 2000, there was an enormous increase of sugar intake in diet worldwide. Processed food—high in carbs, sugar and salt—made with unsaturated and hydrogenated oils along with dangerous trans-fats, entered the food chain. In the new millennium, however, science started taking a sharp U-turn.

The Bitter Truth about Sugar

> *Everything this man said in 1972 was the God's honest truth...every single thing this guy said has come to pass. I am in awe.*
>
> —Professor Robert Lustig on Dr Yudkin

When a 90-minute lecture, 'Sugar: The Bitter Truth', was uploaded by the University of California Television

(UCTV) on 20 July 2009, it instantly went viral.[5] It was heralded as the moment of birth of the anti-sugar movement, for raising the cry for sugar to be treated as a toxin, like alcohol and tobacco. And Professor Lustig of the University of California, San Francisco School of Medicine, who had hailed Dr Yudkin's book as 'prophetic' in his lecture, came to be known as the 'godfather of the sugar tax', for his outspoken campaign that sugar needed to be taxed. By October 2021, the video had garnered almost 14 million views.

Dr Lustig is one of the growing number of scientists who are convinced that sugar is at the root of the waves of non-communicable diseases that afflict the world today. And they are fearlessly speaking out against the sugar industry despite what happened to Dr Yudkin. The anti-sugar brigade features some of the biggest names in nutrition, including Harvard University's Dr Walter Willett, Dr Frank Hu and Dr David Ludwig to Dr Kelly D. Brownell of the Yale School of Public Health.[6] In 2016, Cristin Kearns, assistant professor in the Department of Preventive and Restorative Dental Sciences at the University of California, San Francisco, has uncovered documents to show how the sugar industry—like the tobacco industry—influenced policymakers and academic researchers in the 1960s and 1970s to withhold and manipulate information on the warning signals of heart disease risk linked to sugar (sucrose), while turning dietary fat into a villain.[7]

When Dr Salim Yusuf presented data from a massive study on diet and heart health at the European Society of Cardiology Congress in 2017 (published simultaneously in the *Lancet*), the medical establishment was shocked. The study defied the restrictions and guidelines of long-standing truths on sugar. At the Cardiology Update 2017 symposium, the India-born cardiologist and epidemiologist, who was the former president of the World Heart Federation, expressed clearly what a growing number of scientists and clinicians already felt: 'Every week in the newspaper we read something is good for you. And the same thing next week is bad for you. It's time to clear up the misinformation for good.'[8]

Conducted on more than 150,000 people from 25 countries across five continents, including 29,298 from India, the PURE (Prospective Urban Rural Epidemiology) study has gone against the World Health Organization's (WHO) guidelines that up to 75 per cent of one's daily energy can come from carbohydrates.[9] It has found that a diet high in carbohydrates, in excess of 60 per cent of daily energy, is linked to higher risk of death. The researchers have highlighted foods to eat in moderation: fruits, vegetables, legumes, nuts, dairy, meats/poultry/fish and salt. And foods to avoid are refined grains, processed meat, sugar and sweetened drinks.

More reports are coming out of the PURE study, ongoing for 18 years now. In April 2021, another PURE study found that people consuming a diet in the highest 20 per cent of GI (glycaemic index, the ranking of food based on their effect on blood-sugar levels) have 20 per cent higher risk of heart attack, stroke and death than those who don't.[10] Not all carbohydrates are the same, the report highlights. Most fruits, vegetables, beans and intact whole grains have a low GI, while white bread, rice and potatoes have high GI. Diets high in poor-quality carbs are associated with reduced longevity, while diets rich in high-quality carbs have beneficial effects. As Professor Yusuf, principal investigator of PURE, has pointed out: 'This calls for a fundamental shift in our thinking of what types of diet are likely to be harmful and what types neutral or beneficial.'[11]

Avoid Sugar, I Say

Dr Lustig is investigating all the various names under which the food industry disguises sugar content in food labels, a tactic that makes it extremely difficult for the common consumer to understand how much sugar they are actually putting into their mouth.[12] Apart from anything that contains 'sugar' on a food label, all the following are actually names of sugar: agave nectar, barley malt, brown rice syrup, buttered syrup, caramel, carob syrup, corn syrup, crystalline fructose, dextran, dextrose, diastatic malt, diastase, ethyl maltol, Florida crystals, fruit juice concentrate, high-fructose corn syrup, malt syrup, maple syrup, Panocha, refiner's syrup, rice syrup, sorghum syrup and treacle. He writes on his website that he has now found at least 300 names for sugar and several hundred more might still exist.[13]

Versatility is the word for sugar: it is hard to think of any other food with such a wide array of properties that lends itself to foods and drinks in so many different ways, that makes the risk of consuming too much—without even being aware of it—so real and whose omission in the diet can bring a world of benefits or inclusion lead to so many disparate diseases. Dr Yudkin's book now reads like a prescient warning:

> Avoid sugar, I say, and you are less likely to become fat, run into nutritional deficiency, have a heart attack, get diabetes or dental decay or a duodenal ulcer, and perhaps you also reduce your chances of getting gout, dermatitis and some forms of cancer, and in general increase your life-span.[14]

3

Blooms, Bees and Sugar, Please

Step out to Bhimbetka to experience man's ancient connection with bees. Forty-five kilometres from Bhopal in Madhya Pradesh, the National Highway 46 leads up to this sprawling rock shelter at the foothills of the mighty Vindhya Range. The meandering Narmada River keeps pace. Palash and Amaltas trees paint the landscape in a riot of bright scarlet and yellow. Dusty-pink foliage of Mahua and lofty Gurjan trees pierce the brilliant blue sky, a reminder of the vast forest that once covered the terrain. The craggy cliffs and rocks tell you the story of a staggeringly ancient human life: bustling hunter-gatherer settlements that thrived here at least 100,000 years ago. Today, the rock shelters house India's oldest, and one of the world's earliest, figurative art.

Along with charging bisons, flying arrows and dancing stick figures, there are quite a few other eye-catching artwork that crowd the smooth sandstone walls. What are they? Look closely and you will see clouds of dots denoting swarms of bees, an abundance of honeycombs hanging from tree branches, humans climbing on ladders to access honey, poking hives with prongs or smoking honeybee colonies. Unanswered questions abound: who painted those and why? What do they tell us about when, where or how the early humans learnt to consume honey, the primordial source of sugar? How important were bees and honey in the diets of these hunter-gatherers that they were etched on caves and rocks? Why did they take great risk to gather honey?

Rewind to 30,000 years ago. Imagine a man creeping down labyrinthine dark caves. He holds, in one hand, a flickering oil lamp to show him the way around the darkness. In his other hand, he holds a little basket of crayons—white, red, green and black—carefully prepared from crushed rocks, plants, spittle and fat. As he deftly balances both, he reaches a roomy chamber, puts down his fire and starts daubing paint on the walls, ceilings, niches and hollows. What did he paint? Nature, stick humans, unreal figures and magical symbols. Before he wraps up for the day, he puts his palm flat against the cave wall and outlines the imprint with paint. His signature, perhaps?

Why did the early man take so much trouble to leave his art in the hidden recesses of dark caves? Startlingly vibrant and energetic, but scholars do not think it was art for art's sake. It was a way of recording daily experiences that made it easier to pass on thoughts and messages: celebrating successful activities, warning about real or imagined dangers, and advocating what mattered most to them. They may have served a magical purpose, too: to communicate with the gods or spirits, pray for protection and prosperity, cast a spell on predators, or control threats and adversities. It is widely believed that the paintings were the work of spiritual leaders and healers, the shaman.[1]

Rock art depicting honey-hunters are common in several prehistoric sites throughout the world. Common to them are the techniques of honey gathering, man–insect confrontation and the role of the shaman indicating the possibility that honey and larvae were an important part of their diet. It seems possible that even at this early stage of cultural development, some kind of religion was practised.[2] In fact, bee and beehive imagery is now recognized as a sacred component of rock art. From Africa, Australia and the Amazon basin to India, bees are depicted as spiritual messengers to the shaman, often along with upside-down floating figures, half-human and half-animal forms and geometrical signs.[3]

In the shadow of the Bhimbetka hills, tribes like Baiga live in small and scattered hamlets. Baiga, India's most primitive and the most vulnerable tribe, draws lineage from a primordial shaman, Nanga Baiga, and is named after him: 'Baiga' means sorcerer. Known for their symbiotic relationship with bees and techniques of collecting honey, they are called in to 'converse' with and 'appease' bees by the state government in case of man–insect confrontations even now. Baiga women, even today, adorn themselves with extensive body tattoo in beehive pattern and celebrate bees with the *Ras Nawa* (ceremonial eating of honey) festival every nine years, to atone for an ancient transgression committed by Nanga Baiga against bees.

Eating against Nature

Far away in time and space, I am on a long-distance telephone call with Dr Devi Prasad Shetty.[4] I am scouting for ideas on the way we eat now, for a special issue of *India Today* magazine. Dr Shetty, one of India's best-known heart surgeons, tosses out a comment that takes me completely by surprise: 'The worst offence against the body is eating against nature.' What exactly does he mean? 'Nature did not want us to eat sugar in its current form,' says the doctor. 'It provided us with fruits, honey and sugar cane. Unfortunately, nature also gave us a somewhat crooked brain, that allowed us to collect honey and process sugar cane, in search of more sugar.'

Just a few sentences, but for me, it has been a flash of insight into what has gone wrong with our food, body, eating culture and the centrality of sugar in it. Dr Shetty is, of course, in a position to make such a judgement. For me, it has taken time (and a lot of research) to understand what he meant. I am now convinced that it's an idea whose time has come: the world is on a slide towards disaster. Our diets are becoming increasingly unhealthy. We eat carbohydrates and sweets in excess, but not enough proteins, fruits and vegetables. We feast on processed foods loaded with refined sugar and empty calories, but few nutrients. We trade off food that is good for health for food that tastes good.[5] While India hurtles ahead as the global hub of diabetes, heart disease and obesity, let's follow Dr Shetty's advice and find out how we are eating against nature.[6]

What exactly does nature intend for us to eat? From

a scientific standpoint, the diet of any species in its natural state is always found to agree with its structure and systems. We are the only species on the planet to eat foods that are not natural to us. There is a growing consensus that our modern diet is not only far inferior to that of our ancestors, it is in fact killing us. The diseases of civilization—diabetes, heart disease and cancers—are spiralling out of control as our nutrition habits go through dramatic changes. Our genome, the blueprint of life that evolved over millennia, however, has not had enough time to adapt. At the centre of this discourse stands sugar. Not the white crystals we know as sugar today, but its original source: honey.

Honeybees and the Early Man

The journey of honey started millions of years ago. Dinosaurs still roamed the earth. The supercontinent of Gondwana that incorporated present-day South America, Africa, Arabia, Madagascar, India, Australia and Antarctica was breaking up and India was a large island drifting northwards. There were no fruits and hardly any flowers in this planet, just great green forests of primitive tree-like plants, closely related to conifers, cycads, ferns, mosses and wild grass. Occasional toothed birds flapped overhead, reptiles slithered around and tiny mouse-sized mammals—our earliest-known ancestors—gnawed on roots and barks. This ancient world changed. Some 130 million years ago, flowers and insects evolved—an accident of genes and nature—to meet each other's needs.

Primitive butterflies with iridescent wings were already fluttering about. Then came the big blooms—water lily, lotus and magnolia—and began changing the way the world looked. Some 130 million years ago, flowers and insects evolved to meet each other's needs. Beetles, flies, butterflies, wasps and bees spread pollens accidentally while feeding on flowers. Evolution helped flowering plants become the most successful of all plants. To attract the buzzing pollinators, flowers started developing alluring colour, scent, shape, and sugar-rich nectar and pollens. Bees proved to be the masters at gathering nectar and pollen in the insect world.[7] They provided ancient humans their first sweet treat: honey.

A New Source of Energy Appears

An unusual diet narrative plays out across millennia, as archaeologists discover new fossils of our distant human ancestors, collectively known as *hominin*. Here's how: six million years ago, humans are found eating fruits, leaves, bark, seeds, nuts, roots, tubers and insects, much like chimpanzees, gorillas and bonobos, our closest relatives in the animal kingdom. Around 300,000 years ago, as a climate shift started to dry up forests, a new source of energy appeared on the ancient platter, point out researchers working at the interface of anthropology, nutrition and evolutionary theory. The earliest-known modern human, *Homo sapiens*, had rounder, bigger brains that helped them develop tools, language, self-awareness and, perhaps, the modern diet. The honeybee originated in Asia and spread to Africa and Europe around this time.[8]

What is the new source of energy in the proto-modern diet? The answer to that question again links up to the big debate: what is our natural diet? Conventionally, it is believed to be meat and marrow, often scavenged from the leftovers of large carnivores—lions to sabre-toothed cats—that became the new source of micro- and macronutrients and led to our large brains.[9] Others say, it's not meat: carbohydrate-dense vegetables sourced from roots, tubers, rhizomes and underground stems allowed for brain expansion. Higher carbohydrates may lack sugar but are rich in starch and fibre. Yet another hypothesis points out, evolution adapted our ancestors genetically to cope with sugar in diluted forms, available abundantly in fresh fruits. Undiluted sugar and dietary salt, which accelerate the absorption of sugars, were unknown to prehistoric humans. The diluted sugar best preserved their blood glucose response.[10]

How does the evidence stack up? The spotlight is on human anatomy and physiology: unlike carnivores, we have small, blunt teeth, with stub-like canines and small molars, a small mouth and mobile jaws, which don't favour tearing into raw hide and flesh. We chew our food with the help of digesting enzymes in our saliva, while carnivorous animals simply bite off chunks of meat and swallow them whole. Our hands don't end in sharp claws, our nails are soft and fingers are perfect for picking up fruits. Our long, coiled digestive system makes for slow digestion, whereas carnivores have short digestive tracts and fast digestion. Our livers have very limited capacity to remove cholesterol (found only in animal foods).[11] In other words, through millions of years of evolution, the human body has evolved for plant-based diets, although we have managed to thrive by finding meals to suit us in any environment, through adverse climatic and ecological conditions.

Cereals in diet is undoubtedly an important step in human evolution, but it comes much later—120,000 years through to 65,000 years ago—when our ancestors are found roasting and eating plant starches from tubers and rhizomes, as reflected in charred food remains from hearths discovered at the Klasies River Cave in South Africa.[12] About 78,000 years ago, their diets were varied, rich with 55 types of seasonal plants, nuts, fruits, seeds and vegetables, as shown by the excavations at Gesher Benot Ya'aqov in Israel. With improving environmental conditions some 50,000 years ago, the hunter-gatherers moved towards the creation of cereal-based meals by grinding, sieving, kneading and cooking wild einkorn wheat, barley and oat grains into flatbreads, the essential food for most people even today.[13]

An influential hypothesis comes from Harvard primatologist Richard Wrangham.[14] He argues that the shift from raw to processed foods—or the invention of cooking about 300,000 to 400,000 years ago—has given rise to the modern man (*Homo erectus*) and ultimately the crisis we face now. Cooked food is soft, energy-rich, faster to eat, simpler to break down in the gut and easier to absorb more calories than raw food. It has allowed the early humans to extract more fuel to build bigger brains and body size. More productive activities such as developing tools, agriculture and social networks have followed. In fact, it is the innate human knack for innovative food processing that has made us victims of our own success in modern times: our diets increasingly give us more calories than we can burn.

The latest strand in this body of discourse suggests honey as a crucial food behind the story of human evolution.[15] One of the most energy-dense foods in nature, honey contains 80–95 per cent sugar, yet is easy to digest. Honey also contains trace amounts of several essential vitamins, minerals and antioxidants. The ability to break open beehives and collect honey may have given the early humans a nutritional edge over other species. The commercially produced liquid honey may have small amounts of protein, but wild honey with traces of bee larvae make for high-quality food source of fat, protein, essential minerals and B Vitamins. To researchers, it may have provided critical energy to fuel one of our most expensive organs, the brain, which accounts for just 2 per cent of body weight but needs the maximum share of blood flow from the heart, oxygen and sugar uptake of the body.

Humanity's Most Sweeping Innovation

The invention of cuneiform writing some 6,000 years ago in Iraq is conventionally taken as the point of transition from prehistory to history. In the journey of sugar, however, the historic era begins long before, with the appearance of the first farmers some 10,000–12,000 years ago. The agricultural revolution—humanity's most sweeping innovation which came about with the domestication of animals—has produced the kind of society in which most of us live today and provided the economic basis for the rise of cities and states, trade and technology, culture and recreation. The shift from foraging to farming, however, has brought down the variety of nutrients in our diet. Archaeological digs of the world's earliest-known farmers at Tell Abu Hureyra in modern Syria record a drop from over 150 wild plants to just a handful of crops in the diet. The ancient diet was no longer a balanced combination of carbohydrates with protein and fats from nuts, seeds, shellfish, fish, and small and large fauna.

The exploitation of bees, however, continued unabated as a sweetener and for various technological, ritual, cosmetic and medicinal applications for the last 9,000 years, say scholars.[16] Honeycomb patterns joined ancient civilizations, from Çatalhöyük in Turkey 9,000 years ago to the expansive civilization that developed in the Indus-Ghaggar-Hakra river valley from around 8,000 years ago. Honeycomb patterns and motifs were everywhere: from town planning and house designs, to pottery and ornaments. Bees appeared on seals too. From remains found in excavations at Mohenjo-Daro and Harappa, both thriving centres of commerce, it is surmised that traders dealt in gold, metalwork, pickled fruits, vegetables, wine and honey. At an Indus food exhibition curated by the National Museum at Delhi in February 2020, the sweet treats displayed and served were bars of puffed rice and flaxseed tossed in honey, like *chikki*, the healthy snack that's still prepared in India.

The Obsession with Madhu

In the Vedic age, honey turned into a metaphor for all things sweet and light. The earliest sacred hymnal of India, the Rig Veda (1500 BC) mentioned *madhu*, the Sanskrit word for honey, over 300 times—not just for eating or anointing. It was sweetness itself, *madhura*, the favourite of the gods, and everything that was pure and blessed; the sweetest metre in prosody, *madhucchanda;* the secret essence of the Vedas, *madhu-vidya;* and one of the five nectars of the gods, *pañcāmṛta*. The Rig Veda called for peace on earth by invoking honeyed winds, rivers, trees, animals, nights, days, the dust of the earth and the heavens. Honey was the first sweet used by humans and even after sugar cane entered the Indian diet, the idea of madhu continued to exert its influence. Even Krishna was depicted sometimes as a blue bee, drinking the nectar of a divine lotus.

The earliest reference of sugar cane appeared in the Atharva Veda (2000–1400 BCE): the cultivation and crushing of *ikshu* into jaggery or guda (gur). Dark brown and gritty, *sarkara,* the parent word for sugar in Sanskrit, did not seem to have the appeal of the thick, golden fluid produced by industrious bees. Madhu continued to be the mainstay of culinary art, *pakasastra;* the sweet drink of *madhuparka* (curd, honey and ghee) was offered to guests; it was the remedy for indigestion in Ayurveda and the key element in the ancient restorer, *cyavanaprasa,* to boost immunity. It was also the route to one's last rites, *piṇḍa daan*. In 321 BCE, Kautilya's *Arthasastra* repeatedly mentioned madhu as a simile, even for sweet grape juice.

In the Mahabharata (200 BCE), King Yudishtira fed 10,000 scholars *payasam*, the same word that is used even now, prepared with rice, milk, honey and also fruits and roots.[17] Centuries after sugar displaced honey, the word 'madhu' remained in India's collective consciousness as a name, for both women and men.

Reed of Honey without Bees

How did the wild sugar cane grass become a source of sugar? It could have originated in Northeast India and Bengal, at Papua New Guinea or Southeast Asia.[18] It was indigenous to India and the Indus people possibly used it as fodder for domestic animals. Around 6000 BCE, people in New Guinea began to cultivate sugar cane, chewing and sucking on the stalks to drink the sweet juice within. The processing of that sweet juice into sugar was invented in India. By 500 BCE, Indians knew how to turn bowls of the tropical grass juice into crude crystals of sugar. The 'reed that produces honey without bees', was the famous comment of Nearchos, an army officer of Alexander of Macedonia, as the Greeks made their first acquaintance of India in 327 BCE. It was not just sugar, the Greeks were also amazed at the spectacular consumption of honey by Indians. Alexander's historian Aristoboulos wrote about honey being 'exposed for sale in great quantity'.[19] Sugar travelled with traders and Buddhist monks to China, Persia, Northern Africa, and eventually to Europe in the eleventh century.

The perilous effect of sugar was first mentioned in a 3,500-year-old papyrus procured by German egyptologist

Georg Ebers. The 20-metre-long scroll was among the oldest preserved medical documents, dating back to Pharaoh Amenhotep I. It provided a rare insight into the early practice of medicine. The papyrus was hailed as the first known medical reference to diabetes, but the phrase—'to eliminate urine which is too *asha*'—was unclear and could mean both 'plentiful' and 'often'. Did it mean diabetes, a urinary tract infection or cystitis?[20] How could diabetes afflict a society where sugar cane was unknown and honey was too scarce and expensive to be a major factor? The word 'diabetes' was used first by the Greeks to describe a medical condition where large amounts of water were consumed and urine produced. The Romans added the term 'mellitus', meaning 'sweet as honey', to denote urine that was sweet.

The symptoms of diabetes started appearing in India from the second millennium BCE. The Atharva Veda, which first mentioned ikshu, was also the first to refer to symptoms we now associate with diabetes, *asrava* (morbid flow). The key symptoms were identified: thirst, excretion of sweet urine and loss of weight. The names given to the disease were a variation on the same theme, unusual urination, which possibly startled them the most: *prameha* (to flow), *madhumeha* (honey urine) and *mutrasrava* (excessive urination). There was also recognition of the role played by sugar cane. A hymn in the Kausika Sutra of Atharva Veda went: 'As between both heaven and earth stands the *tejana* (fragrant grass), so let the *munja* (sugar cane) stand between both the disease and the flux (*asrava*).'[21]

Indian texts before the Common Era chronicled

polyuria: unusual, excessive amounts of urine or urine that attracted ants. Of the seven common diseases recorded by early Buddhist texts (fourth–fifth century BCE), almost all were infections. *Madhumehika* (honey urine) was the only lifestyle disorder that manifested without painful symptoms. It was also the only disease that was called 'high', possibly indicating an affliction of the rich. The inimitable Kautilya, who assisted the first Mauryan emperor Chandragupta in his rise to power, penned in his book of advice, *Arthashastra*, how to injure an enemy by making them victims of diabetes. Evidently, madhumeha was not just about unusual micturition, it was widespread and recognized as an incurable and dangerous disease.[22]

What about the medical masters of the ancient world, who created the living tradition of Ayurveda, the science of life and longevity that Indians still abide by? The medical treatises of Charaka and Susruta of the first millennium BCE diagnosed by these symptoms: when urine tasted like honey, was silky to the touch and attracted ants. Sweetness appeared not only in urine but the whole body and led to the derangement of metabolism (*dhatu paka vikriti*).[23] The ancient masters factored in overnutrition and lack of exercise as a cause of the disease: a couch-potato lifestyle and addiction to meat, milk products, new grains, drinks and food made of sugar and jaggery—a combination that enhanced mucous (*kapha dosha*) in the body. The key aberrations were *mithyaharavihara* (improper dietary habits and lifestyle) and foods with sweet taste, *madhura rasa*.

Charaka provided a unique insight into diabetes in India: excessive consumption of *havis*, or the sacred food offered as oblation during sacrificial rites (*yagnya*) to propitiate the gods. Havis entailed a lavish spread of carbohydrates and fats: grains, milk, ghee, honey, sugar, leaves, plants and seeds. With 80,000 out of a lakh hymns of the four Vedas dedicated to listing rituals, ceremonies and actions, yagnya had always been the backbone of the Aryan society. Increasingly, however, it had become elaborate, complicated and expensive, finely woven into the caste hierarchy. There were rituals for every occasion, big and small, covering all aspects of human needs and desires. Indeed, as has been said, 'The life of an Aryan was a series of sacrifices performed under the supervision of the *Brahmana* priests.'[24]

Crystalline sugar spread from India along caravan routes to the early Islamic worlds of North Africa. It was treated as a spice and charged prohibitively by the merchants.[25] It reached the Mediterranean in the thirteenth century and by the late fifteenth century, sugar was being consumed by European elites: a pound of sugar cost more than three days' wages of a skilled craftsman in England.[26] There was a growing demand, but trade routes were dangerous and local tariffs expensive. The search for a way out led to sponsored exploratory expeditions and the discovery of new water routes to China and India. New trade routes eventually led to European colonialist expansion, claim over land, resources and highly exploitative labour practices.[27] Slave-based sugar cane plantation economies in Brazil, the Caribbean, Cuba and the American South led to the growth of the sugar industry to feed Europe's love for sugar.

Rise and Rise of Modern Sugar

The year 2021 marks 100 years of the discovery of insulin by a team of Canadian doctors: Frederick Banting, Charles Best, John Macleod and James Collip. A scientific milestone, insulin has been a lifesaver for millions ever since. Insulin is central to the treatment of diabetes. People with type 1 diabetes, who cannot produce the insulin hormone in their body, are able to live long and well. And for people with type 2 diabetes, who cannot use sugar in their blood efficiently, it has been a blessing. Today, at least 200 million people around the world need insulin. With both type 1 and type 2 diabetes on the rise, the demand for insulin is on a steep incline. A Stanford University study predicts that insulin demand to treat just type 2 diabetes will go up by over 20 per cent from 2018 to 2030. The journey of insulin, however, has not been smooth.[28]

From the eighteenth century, science rallied in support of sugar demand. With steam-powered sugar mills, the production of sugar became increasingly mechanized. At the very heart of scientific endeavour, however, was chemistry. By the mid-nineteenth century, scientists across Europe had figured out the fundamentals of sugar: the sweet carbohydrate in sugar cane (sucrose) was different from honey, but similar to sugar beet; the carbohydrate in grapes was also different from cane sugar but identical to honey (glucose); honey contained a third kind of sugar (fructose). European chemists, especially in Germany, were finding out about all types of carbohydrates: lactose (milk and milk products), mannose (legumes), ribose (meat and seafood), maltose (malted products and germinating cereals), starch (cereal grains, unripe fruits, vegetables, legumes and tubers) and cellulose (fruit skins, seeds, shells, vegetable stalks and leaves).

Thanks to Matthew Dobson, an English physician and experimental physiologist, in the course of the investigation, it was found that excess sugar stored in the liver appeared as glucose in blood and urine. He also observed two types of diabetes: type 1 and type 2. John Rollo, a Scottish military surgeon, was the first to treat a patient with low-carbohydrate, high-fat and high-protein diet, thus beginning the modern dietary approach to prevention, management and potential remission of type 2 diabetes. In the 1800s, French physiologist, Claude Bernard, discovered that sugar in the urine of diabetics comes from the liver, where it is stored and provides the body with a readily available source of energy if blood glucose levels fall. He coined a name for the stored sugar—'glycogen'.

Before Dr Banting and his colleagues at the University of Toronto isolated insulin, people with diabetes did not live long; there wasn't much doctors could do for them. The most effective treatment was to put patients with diabetes on very strict diets with minimal carbohydrate intake. This could buy patients a few extra years but couldn't save them. Harsh diets (some prescribed as little as 450 calories a day) sometimes even caused patients to die of starvation. Doctors tried to treat diabetes with high doses of salicylates, a group of aspirin-like compounds, and even morphine and heroin. The salicylates reduced sugar levels, but at a cost: side effects included constant ringing in the ears, headaches and dizziness.

The last century has witnessed continuous innovation: from the early clunky syringes with large-bore needles to insulin pumps in the 1970s, from insulin pens in the 1990s to sensor-augmented smart pumps that closely mimic the human pancreas in 2006, from artificial pancreas in 2015 to bionic pancreas in 2017—the journey of innovation continues. At the cutting edge of research, there are the smart insulins and smart patches, micro-needles and artificial intelligence devices that promise to transform the field. Between Dr Banting, who received the Nobel Prize in 1923, and Yoshinori Ohsumi, the Japanese scientist who won the 2016 Nobel for his work on autophagy (harnessing the body's own biology to prevent and treat diseases like diabetes), over 30 scientists have won the Nobel Prize for their work on diabetes in the last 100 years.

Yet, the sugar disease is still not curable; it is still rising exponentially across the world. Today's treatments may be more effective, safer and gentler but continue to be out of reach of millions because of high pricing and the complicated regimen of injections and finger pricks to monitor blood sugar. There are just three manufacturers of insulin who decide its price today. In the past 15 years, insulin prices have tripled. Although the discoverers wanted insulin to be affordable to even the poorest sufferers of diabetes, a 100 years later it is still inaccessible to tens of millions of people worldwide. It will be wiser to remember the build-up of our knowledge of food and eating over the centuries, and in the case of sugar, over millennia. It is said, diseases are the results of complex interactions between our genes and culture.[29] So, ignore your evolutionary past at your peril.

4

Sweet Cravings of a Stone Age Brain

Imagine a day, some two million years ago. A man wakes up from sleep. As the early morning sun begins to soar high on the African skies, he steps out of his cave to watch the horizon. He is hungry, his stomach growls. He yanks a stem from the grassy field and bites into it, then stops mid-chew: a sweet aroma is blowing in the wind. It's a fragrance that beckons him, away from his daily diet of grasses, sedges, worms, grasshoppers and occasional tiger nuts. 'Mmm, sweet,' he thinks and ambles off in search of some sugar rush.

In the forest, at the edge of the open grassland, he finds a tree with a dense canopy and hundreds of fruits—yellow, pink, red and purple—strung out on its wide-spreading branches. He climbs up, smells, touches and squeezes the fruits, just as you would shop for fruits in the market today.[1] He bites into those that look sweet: red, soft and squishy. He devours as many as he can, before rushing back to his shadowy lair. He has to share with his cave mates the story of his latest find, a tree with sweet fruits, before roving hordes of giant baboons descend and loot.[2]

He is your ancestor, called *Paranthropus boisei* by paleontologists and fondly the 'Nutcracker Man' for his massive teeth, triple the size of the modern man's.[3] Discovered in the 'Cradle of Mankind', between the Olduvai Gorge and the Tugen Hills of Tanzania in Eastern Africa, his fossil remains reveal today that he was a young man who roamed the savannas in the distant past.[4] Dental microwear texture analysis of his ancient teeth uncovers what he ate in the days before his death: sweet and juicy fruits, like the fig.[5]

A Brain Built on Sugar

The Nutcracker Man lived in a world where food was limited. Foraging fruits from tall trees was tough, no food was grown and little could be stored. Sugar cane was still a giant tropical grass, harvesting honey was an occasional treat, and hunting was irregular and dangerous. Our forebears struggled every day to avoid starvation. Yet, from around this time, between two million and 500,000 years ago, the transformation towards modern humans took off: height and weight increased, teeth and gut became smaller and, most importantly, a doubling of cranial capacity indicated a significant increase in brain size. What was going on?

It is a puzzle that has led researchers to seek a better understanding of the foods eaten during key stages of evolution. The long-standing argument has been that our ancestors transitioned to meat-eating and the protein surge made a bigger brain and body possible. The evolution of human characteristics, including the ability to colonize varied environments, was the result of this ecological adaptability and those who could not adapt perished. Think of the Nutcracker Man and his people: they are likely to have met with an evolutionary dead end, because they failed to make a transition from a plant-based diet to a meat-based diet at a time of food scarcity and became extinct.

This argument has now turned upside down. It is now believed that sugar—not meat—has been the prime source of fuel for our bigger brains, changing anatomy and faster mating strategies in the last 4.4 million years. Meat may have been a preferred food for our ancestors, but the amount of energy requirement humans can derive from proteins has a limit, then as now. Protein poisoning occurs when the body takes in too much protein for a long period of time. Excessive protein intake (greater than 35 per cent of the total calories one eats) can put the body at risk of toxic levels of ammonia, urea and amino acids in the blood.

Sugar, on the contrary, can be rapidly digested and converted to energy in the body.[6] It can also be stored in the body as fat and must have provided energy during lean periods of food scarcity. In the course of evolution, the human brain has become almost five times larger, with blood flow rate growing more than nine times. It is argued that the large human brain needed more energy, 20 times more than any other organ.

What is the source of sugar that led to bigger brains? To some, it is the fig, a particularly sugar-rich and nutritious fruit.[7] A large number of fossils of our early human ancestors have been found with fig remains in the crevices of their teeth. Fig is one of the first fruits to be domesticated as nomadic hunter-gatherers shifted to a sedentary lifestyle. The dawn of agriculture is believed to have come with the fig tree some 11,000 years ago in the Lower Jordan Valley—long before wheat, barley and legumes were farmed.[8] Figs are deeply linked to the rise of religion: it is the first fruit tree mentioned in the Bible, the Tree of Life the Egyptian Pharaohs built their graves with, the tree under which the Buddha attained enlightenment and the tree Krishna identified with in the Bhagavad Gita: 'Of all trees, I am the holy fig tree.'

New research, however, questions the ability of figs, fruits and berries to supply enough energy required for the growth of large human brains. Most fruits are available seasonally. And uncultivated fruits are typically not as rich in sugars as those obtained from modern domesticated varieties. Even today, berries typically contain only 3–4 grams sugars per 100 grams edible portion and would need to be eaten in huge quantities per day. Fruits and berries may have supplemented the early human diet by providing essential vitamins and micronutrients but are unlikely to have fulfilled consistent energy requirements of their large brain.

It is now believed that a high carbohydrate diet has been an important evolutionary force for humans. Researchers posit that plant carbohydrates, especially starches stored by plants in the form of underground tubers and bulbs—basically, wild versions of modern-day foods like carrots, potatoes and onions—have been an essential dietary component to meet the demands of an enlarged brain, to support increased lung capacity as well as successful reproduction. Compared with primates, humans have many more copies of the gene essential for breaking down calorie-rich starches. Even today, 50–70 per cent calories in our diet come from starch alone.[9]

This would not have been possible without the widespread and controlled use of fire for cooking food, a trait found only in humans. Raw foods do not supply sufficient calories: many plant foods are too fibre-rich when raw, while raw meat is too tough to allow easy chewing.[10] Although the timing of widespread cooking is not known, it is believed cooking led to changes in digestive anatomy seen as early as 1.8 million years ago: first, by enhancing the ability of early humans to exploit starch-rich underground roots, tubers, corms and rhizomes, seeds, certain fruits, nuts and inner barks of some trees in their diet; second, cooking made food tender, soft enough for infants, more diverse and enjoyable.

Starch digestion is believed to have enhanced the availability of dietary sugar to our ancestors, greatly increasing the energy supply to the brain, lungs and red blood cells—accelerating an increase in the brain size. Cooking can also be expected to have increased dietary intake to meet additional daily energy expenditure, with far-reaching effects, like bipedality, social behaviour, higher reproductive rates and increased body size, especially of females and infants. Scholars propose that postmenopausal females played a central role in foraging for starch-rich food and food sharing, enabling younger females to reproduce more frequently. Meat has possibly formed an irregular component of their diet, with hunting as much to do with status as nutrition—as seen in chimpanzees.

The Primordial Taste

Taste signals nutrients in food. Of the five different tastes distinguished so far—sweet, bitter, salty, sour and umami—sweet taste plays a central role. For us, it's a primordial taste, linking us to our ancient past, even to the days of the dinosaurs. Like most mammals, we detect sugar molecules with a sensor in our taste buds. It's an adaptive mechanism, because this sensor doesn't work for all in the animal kingdom. Animals that depend on blood and meat wholly do not get sugar and do not need the sweet taste.[11] For instance, carnivorous dinosaurs lost their ability to taste sugar and their progeny, modern birds, mostly live on insects and grains and do not have the ability to taste sugar. Lions, tigers, hyenas, seals, dolphins, vampire bats and even cats have a faulty sugar sensor and can't taste sugar.[12]

Why do humans have this taste? It is believed, we have evolved it as a mechanism for survival. Our body needs energy from food to survive and thrive. We get this energy from glucose, a simple form of sugar. For every cell in the body, glucose is the main source of energy. And our brain, so rich in nerve cells, needs the most energy and demands the most sugar. In fact, the brain can't do without sugar. Thinking, memory and learning, all are closely linked to sugar levels and how efficiently the brain uses this fuel. The story of sugar is deeply linked to the brain.

The sweet taste has been adaptive in other ways, too. Scholars have shown that it has been a survival pathway for us, and many other species, especially during adverse planetary conditions. It can be said that early earth was an inhospitable terrain.[13] In the last half a billion years, there have been at least 18 mass extinctions—from volcanic eruptions, glacier movement and changes in atmospheric gases, to fluctuations in global temperatures and asteroid impacts. Mass extinctions have occurred frequently, about five of which wiped out 75 per cent of species globally. The species that survived have developed remarkable means of survival.[14]

One of the most important means of survival in adverse conditions is to have sufficient food, water, minerals, electrolytes, nutrients and oxygen levels to maintain bodily functions. For many species, including humans, the key has been to create and store caches in the body itself. We have done this by enhancing the activity of sugar in our body. A simple sugar found in the body is fructose, derived primarily from fruits and honey. Fructose can shift the body towards storing fuel as fat and glycogen, the sugar stored primarily in the cells of the liver and skeletal muscle for a quick boost of energy or when the body is not getting sugar from food. This fuel store can be used to provide energy and water at a later date.

Fructose causes salt retention and raises blood pressure—likely to help survival if dehydration or salt deprivation sets in. Fructose can also change the pathway by which sugar is transformed into energy, thereby bringing down oxygen demands in situations where oxygen availability is low.[15] It is believed that at least twice in the history of species, the activity of fructose to generate fat occurred during periods of mass extinction: first, 65 million years ago, when three-quarters of the plant and animal species on earth were destroyed, including the dinosaurs, due to a major asteroid impact; and the second, about 12–14 million years ago, when changes in global ocean chemistry led to mass destruction of marine animals.

There is more to the story. Millions of years of evolution have made sure that your brain rewards you every time you eat sugar, because that act is fundamental to your survival. And pleasure is the brain's way of rewarding you. Your brain has pleasure hotspots that light up the moment you come across sugary treats, because sugar has many ways to activate this circuitry.[16] For long, neuroscientists have believed that dopamine, the brain chemical that controls feelings of well-being, amps up the pleasure circuit. From the 1980s, lab experiments have shown that there is more to the story and sugar plays a central role in this. For instance, lab rats on dopamine suppressants still lick their lips—a sign of enjoyment—when drinking sugar water.[17] Scientists now say, when it comes to sugar, our brain has an especially strong dopamine response. We keep liking and wanting more sugar to get the dopamine effect.[18]

A Powerhouse of Senses

Your brain is smart, it knows how to lure you towards the taste of sweetness. Eyes play a key role in this. We taste first with our eyes, as the proverb goes. It is believed that humans (along with the great apes) have developed colour vision as an evolutionary kick: to detect and select efficiently reddish fruits against the background of green foliage within the forest canopy. The colour red signals high-sugar, high-energy fruits: figs, date palms, apples and berries. Research shows that humans are more motivated by food with more reddish nuances. Is it just a coincidence then that almost every fast-food chain uses the colour red as branding?

The brain primes our eating decisions via sounds, too. When we eat and drink, the tiny bones in our ears vibrate, reaching the brain's pleasure hotspots as electrical impulse that convey food textures: the slurp and squelch of juicy figs, for instance, would have told the Nutcracker Man's brain that they were sweet and fresh. This is the route chefs, marketers and global food companies now take to make their food more desirable for customers. Fizzy drinks companies, for instance, spend months perfecting the sound of cans being opened and poured.

Similarly, smell and flavour stimulate the brain to trigger reward processes. Sweet aromas are powerful appetite cues that are important for food choice, anticipation of food intake and initiation of food intake by steering appetite.[19] There are two types of smell: when you sniff something from a distance, such as the whiff of figs for the Nutcracker Man, you are performing orthonasal smelling. Another kind of smelling occurs when you swallow food (retronasal) and a puff of air gets into your nose. Chemicals that are released from the food as you chew activate the olfactory cells. Soft mouthfeel, as pieces of food churn through the mouth, intensifies the feeling of pleasure.

Science is starting to uncover how all these senses work together to create a perception of food in the brain. A growing body of research is investigating how the background colour of dinnerware may influence taste and flavour perceptions. For instance, exactly the same dessert is rated as tasting sweeter and more flavourful when eaten from a white plate rather than a black one. It turns out, food served on round plates are considered 'sweeter' than more angular ones.[20] Again, high-frequency sounds seem to boost the perception of sweetness. Restaurants are now using this science as part of the dining experience: at The Fat Duck restaurant in the UK, for instance, a seafood dish called Sounds of the Sea comes with sand, foam, seaweed, conch shells and headphones—for the diner to hear sounds of waves and seagulls before eating. Neurogastronomy, a term coined by Professor Gordon Murray Shepherd at Yale School of Medicine has emerged as a scientific discipline. Neuroimaging studies are enabling researchers to understand, among other things, how different brands of soft drinks (Coke vs Pepsi) work on different brain networks.[21]

The Craving Brain

Imagine a day in March 2020. A man wakes up to birds singing outside his window and feels disoriented. Everything is deathly quiet: no hustle-bustle on the street below, no honking of horns: 'Uh, oh, it's lockdown time,' he says aloud. He thinks about a tiny virus, no newspapers from this day, his children going online instead of to school ('God only knows what they will learn') and the new idea of working from home. Shops have shut, public gatherings have been cancelled and everybody is staying indoors. He has stockpiled biscuits, laddoos, barfis, soft drinks, jams, chocolate bars, cookies and, of course, beer. But how will he spend his days at home?

Peacefully bored at the very thought, he picks up his mobile, checks his WhatsApp messages, emails and then starts flicking through Instagram sites on food, his latest passion. Someone has posted recipes to use up overripe bananas: 'It's fudgy, super moist and ultra-chocolatey, designed to be eaten as a snack. Grab the recipe and be sure to tag me.' He wonders what his wife might say. He will have to convince her: he has read somewhere that cooking is therapeutic—it boosts self-esteem, quality of life and mood ('Can a banana drink be called cooking?').

The 52-year-old loves food, lots of food, and has a serious sweet tooth. Normally, apart from the three main meals, he consumes endless cups of tea and coffee and snacks through the day—alone, with friends, with family or with guests. His best-loved food hour is after dark, when he trots over to the Jain family's 200-year-old shop near Jama Masjid, at the heart of Old Delhi. He is one among the hungry crowd that throngs the labyrinthine food streets of Chandni Chowk. In the shadow of the Red Fort, as lights twinkle and the tantalizing aromas waft in the air, he joins his friends with a large packet of hot jalebis—to chat, share and soak up the magic of old-world charm.

Across millennia, let's compare the two foodies of their time: the Nutcracker Man, who went looking for food when his stomach grumbled and the middle-aged Delhite, who consumes food until his stomach grumbles. Just think about it: the daily food of the Nutcracker Man must have been about as tasteless as carrots and the food he possibly loved—the sweet fruits and figs—he could barely get enough: two to three figs contain about 13 grams of sugar. We can now say that they gave him dietary fibre and a range of micronutrients. Think of our Delhi foodie: his diet is all about tasty fried sweets. For the pile of jalebi he consumes daily, he needs to walk at 3 miles per hour (mph) for 69 minutes, to burn off about 600 kilocalories (KCal). If you tally up his daily diet, it comes to over 5,000-odd calories, more than double of what is recommended by the National Institute of Nutrition.

If the Nutcracker Man died early (perhaps killed by a predator or in an accident), our foodie has been advised by his doctor to reduce weight and get rid of his belly fat, along with seven kinds of pills every day to treat his diabetes and high blood pressure. Yet, just like his hunter-gatherer ancestor, our foodie is also on a food quest: he has exchanged the forest trail for street food or the grocery store aisle. If his caveman forebear had to make a daily decision on fruits and grasses, he just has to check out new foods, recipes, stalls, stores, restaurants or browse the Internet for food delivery services. What, however, bind him and his prehistoric ancestor are their sweet cravings and hungry brains.

What's happening inside our foodie's brain? Just

above his ears and about an inch-and-a-half inside his head, the horseshoe-shaped hippocampus makes him remember the tasty, crunchy, syrupy ghee-drenched hot jalebi. 'All I want is a jalebi,' he mutters. In each hemisphere of his brain, the caudate nucleus, which influences reward-seeking behaviour and also new habits, is making him salivate over Instagram images. Those images are making his insulin levels spike: his body is ready for the jalebi it thinks it's about to have. Deep inside his brain, flashing images of Chandni Chowk prey on his insula. Just the thought of evenings spent with food and friends feeds into his craving, raising dopamine levels in his brain. 'Some of the best moments of my life,' he smiles to himself. An MRI (magnetic resonance imaging) of his brain would have shown that the parts of his brain involved in food cravings—the hippocampus, caudate and insula—are identical to those involved in drug addiction.

What adds to his sweet craving is that he is a vegetarian. Scientists have shown that protein and fats slow down the release of sugar into the bloodstream.[22] Without those, your blood sugar can rise and fall at an abnormal rate, making your body crave quick energy from sugar. Add stress to it: the coronavirus pandemic has undeniably caused extraordinary stress, anxiety and fear, with an invisible enemy bearing down on the planet. Many a psychologist has advised patients to limit exposure to news and discussions about Covid-19. Stress shoots up levels of cortisol hormone, which, in turn, pushes up sugar levels in the blood, affecting hunger and cravings. And the more the sweet treats, the more sugar boosts serotonin, a brain chemical that regulates mood and makes one feel happier.

He doesn't know that his craving brain is tough on his body. Sugar might be the fuel for cells and the brain, but when taken in excess, it can trigger a cascade of events: a gut hormone, which manages the body's energy balance, goes up in blood, inducing the body to keep eating. The worst sufferer is the hormone insulin, the vehicle by which sugar enters our cells. It sends emergency messages to the cells: 'Mop up all the sugar, use it for energy.' As our foodie continues on his gastronomic journey, his cells, however, defy insulin's commands. Who cares for energy? The foodie is busy filling up the long void of Covid-19-induced boredom with his favourite foods and drinks. He is in a state of blah: sleepy and blissed out, while his body quietly stores all that sugar as fat.

From Pleasure to Peril

How much sugar do you really need in your blood to be healthy and active? Just 4 grams, or slightly less than a teaspoon for a healthy individual weighing about 70 kilograms. That's the measure of sugar circulating in your blood at all times.[23] Your brain needs 20 per cent of it every minute. If sugar comes down to one-fourth teaspoon, the brain shuts down, with fatal consequences. Even a slight change can put your metabolism out of kilter, inviting a host of diseases: a full teaspoon can push you towards pre-diabetes, while a teaspoon and a quarter towards diabetes. The body has evolved a sophisticated control system to protect your sugar levels from swinging up and down. Such brain–body mechanisms have worked well with our Stone Age ancestors, who ate plenty of woody plants and animal meat. But what about now?

Our foods now contain high levels of sugars, fats and salts. Such food was hard to come by in the ancient past, but can now be consumed in great abundance, anytime and anywhere. Some estimates suggest the Paleolithic diet consisted of 1–3 kilograms of sugar per year. Today, the per capita consumption of sugar in India is more than 23 kilograms.[24] It is 66–68.9 kilograms in the US.[25] Processed sugars (which are stripped of vitamins, minerals and fibres), sneaky added sugar and harmful sugary beverages are all over our food chain. All these have been implicated in the steep rise in heart disease, diabetes, hypertension, weight gain, fatty liver disease, stroke and some cancers as leading causes of death worldwide.

Across millennia, what has remained relatively constant is the blueprint of our body: our DNA. But it is now in conflict with our modern lifestyle. Our brain still strategizes to fight against food scarcity and survival. High-energy foods, such as sugars and fats, still stimulate the 'feel-good' chemical dopamine in our brain. The same brain wiring that was meant to reward us with pleasure, now goes out of whack, putting us at risk of irresistible, compulsive overeating—what scientists now call 'hedonic hunger', a powerful desire for food in the absence of any need for it.[26] And we put into disarray our entire system.

Here is one instance of how sugar botches up our carefully regulated brain–body mechanisms: our brains are very good at telling us when to eat and when to stop. At the smell, sight, sound and taste of high-energy food, rich in sugar and fat, a hunger hormone from the stomach increases in the blood. It travels up the blood stream to the appetite centre of the brain, triggering the feeling of hunger, and we start eating. When we have eaten enough, satiety molecules from fat cells in our body trigger the sensation of feeling full in the brain, and we stop eating.

Too much sugar in our blood messes with the crosstalk between the two vital hormones at the appetite centre of our brain: one controlling hunger and the other, satiety. That communication normally makes sure we eat enough and that we don't resort to overeating. If they fail to talk to each other, the appetite centre of the brain does not get the signal: 'stop eating'. Foods rich in sugar and fat trigger hormones in the gut that stop the action of the feeling-full hormone and induces the body to keep eating, ending up with high blood glucose levels in the body.

In the past decade, frontier research in neuroscience has unlocked new secrets of the brain, which shows that the brain is amazingly adaptive: that it can rewire and re-engineer itself, both physically and functionally, throughout life; that it can form new brain cells (neurons) even in adulthood; that the brain can reverse its wiring; that various nerve cells and parts of the brain constantly 'talk' to each other; and that the more brain circuits are used, the more they strengthen—a phenomenon called 'neuroplasticity'.

Neuroplasticity has enabled people to recover from stroke, improve symptoms of autism, and pull out of depression and addictions. Neuroplasticity, however, is a door that swings both ways: bad habits too can get ingrained in the brain. Rewiring can happen in the pleasure circuit. Eating an excessive amount of sugary foods causes the brain to adapt to frequent stimulation, creating a vicious cycle of wanting more sugar and eating more sugar to get the same rewarding kick, exactly like addiction.

The scientific study of pleasure pioneered by Charles Darwin, the naturalist who developed the first scientific theory of evolution, has come full circle.[27] In his 1872 monograph, *The Expression of the Emotions in Man and Animals*, he posits pleasure as an evolutionary response. In the 1950s, the findings of Canadian psychologists James Olds and Peter Milner suggest that they discovered the pleasure centre in the brain. In their lab, rats would repeatedly press levers to receive tiny jolts of current through electrodes implanted deep within their brain.[28] Later, neuroscientists, probing how our food-seeking biology has evolved through millions of years of evolution, call it the 'hedonic hotspots', or brain sites where stimulations amplify sensory pleasure.[29]

The number of books written on evolution, health and disease has increased dramatically in the last two decades. With the epidemic of lifestyle diseases spiralling out of control, the brain, its parts and circuits that encourage consumption of sugar, is getting new attention. New research shows how the modern human body is equipped for problems that most of us do not face any more. As scientists redefine the brain's pleasure circuitry, sugar emerges as the prime culprit in making us eat for the sake of pleasure, rather than for survival. There is a growing consensus that the yearning one experiences—even when the stomach is full but the brain continues to be hungry for sugar—pushes the body towards overeating and lifestyle-induced diseases such as obesity and diabetes.

One of the most lucid exponents, Daniel E. Lieberman, professor and chair of the Department of Human Evolutionary Biology at Harvard University, puts across the paradox of brain and diet of modern humans:

> The food industry has made a fortune because we retain Stone Age bodies that crave sugar but live in a Space Age world in which sugar is cheap and plentiful. Sip by sip and nibble by nibble, more of us gain weight because we can't control normal, deeply rooted urges for a valuable, tasty and once limited resource.[30]

5

What Sugar Really Does to You

Somewhere within the sprawling campus of the All India Institute of Medical Sciences (AIIMS) in Delhi, where patients do not intrude, Dr Nikhil Tandon has his office. You will find the head of the department of endocrinology hunched over his laptop between classes, donning a white coat and a stethoscope, his desk overflowing with papers in depths ranging from a few inches to a foot. Today, he has bad news for me. 'In just over a quarter century, diabetes has shot up by almost 200 per cent in India,' he says as he hands me a document. It's a copy of the research he has conducted with 24 collaborators across the country.[1]

A few years ago, Dr Tandon and his colleagues had changed the conversation on diabetes in India by documenting high blood sugar among schoolchildren. Their investigations in Delhi schools had exposed the flip side of India's growth story: healthy children of urban affluent classes were significantly heavier and had abnormal blood sugar and cholesterol levels. The implications were staggering: clearly, a new generation was growing up with anomalies that could put them in serious danger as adults. His new report was on the hushed but unrelenting assault of sugar in our blood in the last 25 years.

How sugary is our collective blood? Let us count the ways. Diabetes is what Prime Minister Narendra Modi has persistently called the 'biggest threat' we face (in the pre-Covid-19 days); it is what scores of leading politicians suffer from or succumb to; famous faces talk about fighting diabetes and coming out victorious. It is so ubiquitous that matrimonial sites have now added a new category of matchmaking for people with diabetes where they can meet prospective partners with a similar medical history. Even in the courts of law, judges root for healthy food in school canteens. And every day someone, somewhere, buckles under the pressure of crushing hospital bills for having diabetes or any of its complications.[2]

Dr Tandon's report shows a steep rise in the number of people with diabetes: from 26 million in 1990 to over 73 million in 2017. Across every state in the country, diabetes is leading to a cascade of crises: heart disease, strokes, cancers, fatty livers, blindness, amputations, asthma, COPD (chronic obstructive pulmonary disease), kidney disease, tuberculosis, Alzheimer's, dementias, allergies and infections. Twenty-five years ago, diabetes was not even among the top 30 causes of years of life lost (YLL) to premature death and disability in India. Today, however, it is the thirteenth. That's a whole lot of YLL—a calculation health statisticians have begun to use frequently to get the full impact of a disease that is largely invisible.

Used first by the World Bank in the 1990s, YLL means years of lost opportunity and hope: years the sufferers of a disease could have lived if they had not died early or become incapable of enjoying life prematurely. Healthy years lost to diabetes is the highest among all non-communicable, lifestyle diseases in India—a whopping 792, compared with 607 to heart disease, 226 to stroke, 330 to chronic kidney disease, 30 to cancers, 11 to cataract, and 12 to Alzheimer's and dementia. Overweight and obesity, the most important risk factor in diabetes, have seen an out-of-control doubling in the past 25 years. The death rate from diabetes has risen by a benumbing 131 per cent in India.[3]

Diabetes today is globally recognized as the 'largest epidemic in human history'.[4] The disease is progressing at such a fast clip that even projections fail to keep pace: the International Diabetes Federation predicted there would be 324 million people with diabetes globally by 2030, while the WHO estimated 366 million.[5] Diabetes, however, has proved them all wrong: there are already over 463 million adults worldview with diabetes now. The milestone has simply shifted.[6] China, India and the US have the largest numbers and are projected to remain so.

It matters that diabetes is expensive. As a progressive disease, the cost of treatment keeps rising with the years, as more medications are required to control sugar levels. The world faces an economic burden of about $1.3 trillion from diabetes, or 1.8 per cent of global gross domestic product.[7] Medications used to treat diabetes are the most expensive, with insulin prices playing a big part in this. The cost of diabetes medications has zoomed by 58 per cent between 2014 and 2019, nearly double the rate of other drug prices.[8]

In India, diabetes care is largely out of pocket and has been rising exponentially. Studies have repeatedly shown how diabetes contributes to catastrophic health expenditure in low- and middle-income families, wiping out anything between a quarter and one-third of annual incomes.[9] For the higher socio-economic strata, the cost of therapy is almost the same as that in the UK, despite massive differences in purchasing power parity in the two countries.[10] The inexorable and unsustainable rise in cost of care makes diabetes and its complications a killer in every possible way.

Behind the numbers is the reality of an ancient disease that escapes cure in modern times. Scientists are still trying to fit together the puzzle pieces of diabetes, as the coronavirus pandemic has revealed. No other disease allows so much stigma, prejudice or misconceptions. No other disease causes such massive loss in quality of life, personal independence, mobility or mental decline. No other disease hides in hospital records as something else. There is, however, a silver lining to this grim story: an explosion of new research is changing the way diabetes is perceived, understood and treated.

Sugar and the Rebels Within

It all comes down to sugar in the end. Your body needs sugar to keep ticking. Glucose, a simple sugar, is your body's energy currency that your brain and cells use.

When you eat food, huge quantities of digestive enzymes rapidly reduce it to particles of amino acids, sugar and fats. As sugar levels rise in your blood, a flurry of activities starts. Fast-paced conversations—signals, chatters and crosstalks—begin to take place between your pancreas, liver, muscle and fat: how much sugar is present in the blood, how much is to be taken up by cells for fuel, how much should be released from energy stores. That's because sugar is extremely important for your body, but it can't get inside your cells on its own.

Your pancreas—the yellowish-brown, slippery gland, hidden deep in your abdomen—is a bit of a temperamental star. It can get irritated and inflamed easily, giving you diabetes and an expanding girth. But it also does some incredibly important jobs: it generates digestive enzymes, synthesizes opposing hormones insulin and glucagon, and plays a key role in how much and when you should eat or stop eating. Insulin brings down your blood sugar levels, glucagon increases it and together they control, titrate and maintain the sugar level in your blood.

Right after you eat, signals reach your pancreas to release insulin, the hormone that is your body's only key that can open up cells to let the sugar in. As cells absorb sugar, its levels in your bloodstream begin to fall. The pancreas starts making glucagon, the other hormone that signals the liver to start releasing stored sugar. This interplay of insulin and glucagon ensures that cells throughout your body, and especially in the brain, have a steady supply of blood sugar. Inside your cells, the sugar is turned into energy—for you to move, think, breathe, eat and do everything else that you do. Your blood sugar level also returns to the normal between-the-meals range. Perfect.

The problem starts when you have too much sugar in your blood. Maybe, your diet is too rich in polished grains, you consume too many carbs and sugar (think processed food, junk food and soft drinks) or you are overeating. Too much sugar means your cells have to work harder to process the food. Insulin sends urgent messages to your cells: grab sugar out of the bloodstream and use it for energy. If you continue to eat dangerously, your cells stop listening to insulin (you develop what is called 'insulin resistance' in scientific language). Both blood sugar and insulin levels stay high long after eating. Over time, the pancreas gets tired and stops making insulin.

How would you know that your cells and hormones are not doing what they should be doing? Hunger is your cue: you are hungry all the time, but no matter how much you eat, it refuses to subside. Sugar keeps floating in your blood, giving you high blood sugar. You are also tired. Sometimes, you feel as if all your energy has been drained away. You can also lose weight, even though you are eating more than normal, because the excess calories are lost in your urine as sugar now. Excess appetite, thirst and urination are the cardinal symptoms of diabetes.

Glass Half-Full or Half-Empty?

One of the world's oldest maladies, diabetes has proved to be too silent, too sneaky and too stealthy to be conquered even by modern medicine. There is still no cure in sight, but diabetes has caught the world in its grip and struck deep roots in India. The numbers are spiralling beyond control and the sharp toll the disease exacts on finances and quality of life is on the rise. Yet, it is not all gloom: with an explosion of new research and treatments, scientists and physicians espy a silver lining.

Two big ideas dominate the latest thinking on the diabetes front: first, sugar-rich diet and lack of activity determine who develops it, and second, it involves systemic inflammation that affects multiple organs. Scientists are unravelling the complexity of the disease. For instance, until recently, diabetes was considered to be either type 1 or type 2. In the former, which comprises around 10 per cent of the cases, the body's own immune system attacks the cells that produce the hormone insulin. That means, your body can't make insulin and therefore is unable to deliver sugar to your cells. When the body no longer has any insulin-producing cells left, insulin must be injected several times a day—a lifelong process. In type 2 diabetes, which comprises around 90 per cent of the cases, the body produces insulin normally, but cells become resistant to it. Therefore, glucose doesn't reach the cells.

Now scientists say that diabetes is a cluster of separate diseases, with significantly different characteristics. Cluster 1, for instance, is severe and the immune system is at fault. It is broadly the same as type 1 and hits people when they are young and seemingly healthy. The second cluster appears to be very similar to cluster 1, but here the immune system is not at fault. In Cluster 3, although the body makes insulin, it no longer responds to it. Clusters

4 and 5 are milder types of diabetes, the former seen mainly in people who are very overweight and the latter among older people.[11] This raises the hope of providing targeted personalized care, rather than giving everyone the same drug and treatment.

It's an age of possibility for diabetes prevention and treatment. It is the only disease for which maximum drugs are in development. There are currently 11 different categories of medications that work rapidly and in a number of ways to lower blood sugar levels. Newer drugs are appearing every year, which stimulate insulin release and reduce blood sugar without causing low blood sugar, or hypoglycaemia, the bane of treating diabetes. Several of them cause weight loss and have significant salutary effect on heart and kidney disease—the biggest killer in diabetes. There is now a wide array of continuous glucose-monitoring systems—from transdermal patches and sensor implants, to smart insulin delivery systems.

One such candidate scientists are excited about is a hormone released from bone, called osteocalcin, which stimulates insulin secretion in the pancreas. Under scrutiny is the immune system. Researchers have found that fat tissue contains an abnormally large number of immune cells (macrophages) that contribute to chronic, low-grade inflammation: a bodily malfunction that precedes nearly all cases of obesity, type 2 diabetes as well as heart disease. The brain and its role in blood sugar regulation are also being studied. So are hormones from the small intestine, called incretins, which seem to talk directly to the brain and the pancreas in ways that help reduce blood sugar.

Other researchers have shown that free fatty acids (FFA) are an important link between obesity, insulin resistance and type 2 diabetes. FFA levels are elevated in most people who are overweight or obese and they seem to damp down the mechanism by which insulin mediates sugar uptake into cells. At the cutting edge of research is stem cell transplant. Scientists are testing ways to transplant stem cells into people with diabetes, so they can make the insulin they need to control blood glucose levels. Currently, a range of human clinical trials on stem cell research is ongoing and might herald a new age of medicine, where the patient's own stem cells can be used.

An entirely new approach is being adopted for treating the elderly with type 2 diabetes. Doctors are easing up on efforts to achieve strict low blood sugar levels in frailer, older patients, in an approach called de-intensification.[12] The focus is now on reducing overtreatment and balancing benefits and risks with age and illness. High insulin doses often reduce blood sugar levels in the elderly so severely that they tip towards episodes of hypoglycaemia, which may offer few benefits and pose unexpected risks, such as falls and fractures. The Endocrine Society suggests that instead of following strict diabetic diets, older patients with diabetes should eat healthy and limit the intake of simple sugars.

When the Key Goes Missing

He has been bullied since childhood, received unsolicited lectures, censured as a drug addict for taking insulin jabs in public, spent days in hospital intensive care units (ICUs) and faced life-threatening situations. Yet, he has always turned around and fought back, with courage and discipline. His mantra? 'Never give up. Love you zindagi.' All because, Delhi resident Harsh Kohli has type 1 diabetes: his pancreas does not produce insulin.

No one quite knows why some people get type 1 diabetes. Some scientists have linked it to genes, some to viruses (say, rotavirus, the most common cause of severe diarrhoea in infants),[13] some to overactive immune systems that attack the pancreas by mistake and stops insulin, and some to microbes in the digestive tract.[14] The list of possible villains is long: glutens (the protein in wheat which is plentiful in highly processed foods) to microscopic fungi in root vegetables, air pollutants, infant formula feeding and passive smoking.[15]

Whatever the reason, people with type 1 diabetes need lifelong treatment and can slip into fatal conditions from excessive sugar spikes or dips.[16] Their numbers are rising. There are around 1,106,500 million people with type 1 diabetes worldwide.[17] India is the second-largest hub of children with type 1, the first being China. Between monitoring blood sugar and counting calories continuously, keeping a close eye on physical activity levels and carrying insulin jabs, pumps, pens and patches everywhere, what is their life like?

Kohli's life changed one fine day in 1992, when his parents took him to a doctor. He was not even a teenager then, but he was drastically losing weight and he was always tired, always thirsty. The doctor had packed him off to a hospital: he had uncontrolled hyperglycaemia (excessive sugar in his blood). Saline hydrations, insulin drips and injections for 15 days and he was allowed to return home. The hard reality, however, dawned when his mother told him that he could no longer have his favourite chocolates, or any sweets, for that matter.

A new life of daily rituals began. He learnt to push in a needle four times a day, count his carb intake, maintain food logs and listen to his body for sugar cues. He also learnt to ignore the barrage of questions and negative comments from people who did not matter, the teasing and bullying from classmates, the subtle and indirect taunts—for being different. And he took his revenge by focusing on his studies: 'I silenced them all when I became the math topper in school.'

It was in college that the first major incident happened. He suddenly started feeling sweaty, dizzy and shaky.[18] He knew the signs and reached out for a packet of snacks. As he started eating for dear life, a teacher arrived and snatched it away. 'Don't you know eating is not allowed here,' he yelled. The more he tried to explain, the more he got on the wrong side of the college authorities, until he called up his mother. A quiet homemaker, she fought with ferocity and grace to make them understand what having type 1 diabetes meant. The college finally relented, but the experience somehow changed Kohli. College lost its charm.

Kohli can tell you many such stories. And he still battles with his everyday life. A mechanical engineer, he has married the girl he fell in love with in college and is a father to two sons. Life would have been 'perfect', despite the swings between 'hypo' (hypoglycaemia, when blood sugar levels become dangerously low) and 'hyper' (hyperglycaemia, when blood sugar levels go up abnormally), if only his youngest son had not inherited type 1.

He is busy with DIYA (Diabetes India Youth in Action) now. Like him, most of the members have type 1 diabetes. They meet up every now and then, go on treks or cross-country bike rides, collect data and campaign to raise awareness about type 1 and other rare types of diabetes where the pancreas does not produce insulin (such as latent autoimmune diabetes in adults, or LADA). What keeps them going? Just the hope that the future for generation-next will be better than theirs.

The Vulnerable Heart

Right outside Dr Ashok Seth's[19] chamber, there is a silver-framed photograph on a small table. The portrait of a happy, young family of four, laughing into the camera, arms around each other. Seated at the centre is a 30-something man, who once ran for miles, worked out for hours in his personal gym and played badminton at the Siri Fort Sports Complex in Delhi, until he was floored by a sudden heart attack. Dr Seth, chairman and chief cardiologist of the Fortis Escorts Heart Institute in Delhi, looks at the photograph and thinks how different the story would have been now.

Eat healthy, exercise, reduce your weight, check your girth, sleep well, cut down on stress, don't smoke and don't drink: doctors have been sounding out the alarm for years. Diabetes, high cholesterol and high blood pressure are risk factors for heart attacks, along with family history. And even if you are apparently healthy and young, you can be down with sudden cardiac death and disability without warning. The word 'sudden', however, is now being erased out of medical repertoire.

Armed with new research, tests and technology, doctors can now pick up hidden heart problems in astonishing detail. And the villain has changed: from hard plaques (cholesterol-containing deposits) to soft lumps of fat cells that lie silently in arteries, sometimes for decades—until one day they rupture, leading to a heart attack. Called the vulnerable plaque, they are now being blamed for over 70 per cent of sudden heart attacks.

The strangely named plaques can now be captured in advance by the new biochemical markers: high-sensitivity C-reactive protein (hsCRP) in the liver, apolipoprotein (a) in cholesterol and amino acid homocysteine and haemoglobin (HbA1c) in the blood. Each of these biomarkers are linked to diabetes, which has been a well-known risk factor for heart disease, but new scientific developments show how insulin resistance and inflammation drive heart attacks and how low-grade chronic inflammation precedes both diabetes and heart disease.

Take, for instance, the hsCRP, considered the most sensitive predictor of future heart disease. Produced by the liver, these proteins circulate in the blood, their levels rising with infection or inflammation in the body. Elevated levels of hsCRP may predict risk of the first heart attack up to eight to 10 years in advance. Earlier, such patients would have been left alone, but now elevated hsCRP is a cue to start treatment. It has also been linked to an increased risk of future development of diabetes—the hsCRP levels are higher in people with diabetes compared with those without.[20]

When it comes to clogged arteries, the 'bad' LDL cholesterol is still the focus of millions of blood tests. Recent studies have shown that these conventional lipid tests can lead to errors in the assessment of heart attack risk. Replacing them fast are cutting-edge tools that use apolipoproteins (that transport fat and cholesterol in blood), which get altered with diabetes and heart complications. Similarly, homocysteine, a common amino acid in blood, is strongly linked to early development of heart disease and of diabetes. And HbA1c, used increasingly to screen and manage diabetes (the test measures the amount of blood sugar attached to haemoglobin over three months), has been found to predict the risk of heart disease even in people without high blood sugar.

On the Hospital Bed

Both are masterpieces of evolution: one called a 'masterpiece of engineering and a work of art' by one of the world's greatest artists, Leonardo da Vinci;[21] the other described as a 'modest, organized friend, underground worker', by one of the world's greatest poets, Pablo Neruda.[22] The human leg and the liver appear about as different from each other as can be imagined, yet they add up to one story: the story of sugar and what it can do to the human body. They also represent the twin faces of the obesity–diabetes epidemic, the hidden and unexpected collateral damage of a larger war. More than kidney transplant, stroke, heart attack or loss of vision, what puts people with diabetes in the hospital most often are foot and liver complications—largely under-reported, yet two of the gravest fallouts of the sugar disease.

It was on a trip to Vaishno Devi temple in Jammu that 67-year-old Savithri Venkatesh realized how much she valued her feet. She was climbing barefoot up the 4,000-plus steps, when her husband alerted her to the blood-drenched footprints she was leaving on her trail. She was bewildered: she had not felt any pain or burning sensation. Within two years, however, her right toe had to be amputated. It was at the hospital that she met Govind Nahate, 46, a chartered accountant who had no clue as to why white fatty tissues had spread tentacles all across his liver. As baffled as Venkatesh, he had asked his doctor why he never got a hint. It is like that with the liver, he was told.

With 26 bones and 29 joints, held together by a shock absorber ligament, each human foot is serviced by over 7,000 nerve endings. As excess sugar makes the blood heavy, nerves at the periphery of the body remain starved. That makes the feet vulnerable to skin ulcers that can worsen quickly. The inability to feel pressure and sense position leads to imbalance and deformity. The foot remains in contact with the ground for a longer time, changing walking patterns. No amount of antibiotics or dressings can heal this, unless the pressure injury is reduced.

Bad news for Nahate, too: fatty liver disease is rapidly emerging as a health crisis in India. As sugar levels build up in the blood, fat molecules accumulate inside liver cells. The presence of the fattened cells can then lead to inflammation in the liver and damage the surrounding liver tissues. Today, fatty liver damage is being seen in people who do not consume alcohol. That makes it more dangerous. Non-alcoholic fatty liver disease (NAFLD) can stay as a low-grade condition for years. Over time, non-alcoholic steatohepatitis (NASH), a type of NAFLD, damages the liver, changing its structure irreversibly, sometimes leading to cirrhosis, liver failure or even liver cancer.

The Sweet Tooth of Cancer

On 4 February 2021, World Cancer Day, new research made headlines. Conducted over 18 years by the scientists of Imperial College London on 300,000 people with diabetes, it showed that heart disease and stroke were no longer the leading causes of death in people with diabetes in the UK. Between 2000 and 2018, the trend changed, with death by cancer slowly taking over.[23] Did this change mean a link exists between diabetes and cancer? The world of science was shaken to its core.

Nearly a century ago, German biochemist Otto Heinrich Warburg had described the ravenous appetite of cancer cells for sugar. He proposed that cancer cells grow by avidly swallowing up large amounts of sugar from the blood due to a faulty mechanism. Scientists paid no heed. He won the Nobel Prize for Physiology or

Medicine in 1931 for his work on respiration, not cancer. Eventually, his research was dismissed and forgotten. The cancer narrative did not include his ideas, nor were they included in medical textbooks anywhere.[24]

Warburg's theory—called the Warburg effect now—is coming back from the dead. Since the last decade, it has turned into one of the most promising areas of cancer research. Scientists are working across the world to identify what leads a cell to eat more sugar than it should, what role genes and the environment play in this process and, of course, how to slow down or stop tumour growth by starving cancer cells of what they need the most for growth: sugar.[25]

A growing body of evidence shows that type 2 diabetes and cancers share several risk factors: ageing, obesity, diet and physical inactivity, all of which are driven by excessive sugar and insulin in the blood, along with inflammation. The Warburg revival has put the spotlight on insulin. Think of how sugar-heavy diets can elevate insulin levels in blood permanently. In the same way, cancer cells start feeding on sugar when excessive insulin circulates in the blood, when the body's immune system malfunctions, and when there is too much sugar in the blood. Colorectal, pancreatic and breast cancer, for instance, show elevated insulin levels.[26]

Excitement is building around innovative research in the obesity-diabetes-cancer space. New thoughts, new ideas, new methods and new technology are changing scientists' understanding of diabetes and how to attack it. The focus is now on moving research breakthroughs from the lab bench to the patient's bedside.

From Bench to Bank to Bedside

When Jugnu Jain, molecular geneticist, cell biologist and inventor with three patents, returned to India in 2011, after 26 years of pursuing global science, she was stunned to find that India did not have a large-scale national human biobank. India was groaning under non-communicable diseases like diabetes, yet without a biobank how could government policies be driven by data and lab research reach the Indian patient's bedside? Even China had strong biobanks: if China could do it, why couldn't India? With that thought, she set up Sapien Biosciences in 2012, headquartered in Hyderabad: the country's first pan-India and commercial biobank.

Jain specializes in diabetes, cancer and immunology. She studied genetics at G.B. Pant University of Agriculture and Technology, Uttarakhand, at a time when female students were not encouraged or given much consideration. The joy of unlocking the secrets of genes has made her play for global science at institutes of excellence—University of Cambridge, UK, and Harvard Medical School, US—to learn from the best of teachers. The excitement of discovering genetic defects in the blueprint of one's body and taking proactive measures to stem the consequences have led her to work with the US biotech firm, Vertex Pharmaceuticals, known for its transformative medicines for life-threatening diseases.

But what are biobanks? For every disease, there are infinite unanswered questions: why do some people get certain symptoms and complications early on while others don't; who is at greater risk and who is not; who should be given what treatment. Biobanks are a repository of tissues, blood, urine and other bodily fluids, leftover from surgery or diagnostic procedures, from which researchers can gather such data and gain insight into the genetic and molecular basis of diseases in a particular population. Results from biobank studies can boost, sometimes even replace, the need to test new drugs.

An acute problem in a country like India is that most new, life-saving drugs need a very expensive manufacturing process, something that is affordable in affluent countries. India makes copies of drugs, although the generic drugs do not work the same way on the Indian population, given the difference is structure, genes and other biological attributes. India also does not have large-scale population studies on Indian tissues to understand the risk factors for diseases Indians typically suffer from, where, at what age or the treatments needed. Jain is determined to help manufacture original drugs with such granular data, produced with Indian research.

'Jugnu Jain has been changing the landscape of biobanking in India. Sapien Biosciences has emerged as India's first central biobank predominantly upcycling medical waste for R&D of new diagnostics, drugs, and reagents.' In 2020, Jain received that citation along with a 'Women Transforming India' award from NITI Aayog, the Government of India's premier think tank. The road ahead may be long and uphill for people like her, but it is the new way of doing science—from laboratory bench to bedside—that promises to fast-track biomedical advances in the service of patient benefit, especially in complex diseases like diabetes.

6

Sugar and the Slow Burn

> Sit relaxed. Tune in to the world around you: the aroma of trees, the musky scent of the earth, the rustle of leaves, the crunch of twigs, the whipping of wind through tall grass. Feel the cool depth of the forest. Absorb the colours of nature: the flowers, the berries, the birds, the snail shells. Watch the ferns. They are the oldest plants on planet earth. They know how to survive. Breathe in the crisp, clean air. Count to four as you breathe in. Pause. Count to five as you breathe out…

The trainer uses a soothing monotone as he asks us to soak up the energy of nature with our five senses. It's a forest therapy session in progress: a bit of mindfulness, a bit of Japanese *shinrin-yoku* 'forest bathing' and a lot of controlled breathing. Hidden from the public eye, at the foot of an extinct volcano, here, silence stretches over hundreds of acres. Gigantic trees pillar the green void. Dirt roads lead up to little prayer shrines. Scattered at a distance are villas with glass floors and see-through walls, swimming pools that edge into waterfalls, tree houses with open-air showers, raw-food restaurants and sprawling organic farms.

It's a refuge for anyone who seeks a break, respects the outdoors and thinks of nature as medicine. Here, ancient healing traditions meet modern science. Immersive experience of nature promises to enhance well-being, bring down stress and cortisol levels in the blood and soothe the natural killer cells of overactive immune systems. People come here to rest, reboot and reverse the hidden slow burn of modern times, chronic inflammation—be it from stress, ageing, pollution or the ubiquitous ravages of sugar in the modern diet.

How do they know they have inflammation? Some have the diseases that go with it: heart disease and diabetes to cancer. Others complain of perennial fatigue, burnout and insomnia, frequent infections and allergies, anger, mood swings and panic attacks. They talk about intense cravings for sweet-laden, calorie-rich food, which don't bring satisfaction yet add to weight. And, they come here in search of something: to align their system for optimum vitality and wellness.

In a Drop of Blood

A therapist pricks my finger for a drop of blood. She prepares a smear and mounts it on a high-powered microscope. Seconds later, millions of soap bubbles float across a computer screen. They are my red blood cells, swimming in plasma serum and ferrying oxygen to my tissues. Call it the mystery of my life: my 'blood picture'. If most of the bubbles are round and free-floating,

I don't need to worry. If they clump together and look pointy or squashed, it would mean that my cells are suffering from oxidative stress—the sure-fire path to inflammation.

What is oxidative stress? 'It's a condition when your body can't get rid of toxic oxygen molecules, called free radicals,' the therapist explains. 'Free radicals: that sounds nice, but why should I have toxic oxygen molecules in my body?' I ask. 'Everybody does,' the therapist says. 'All the normal processes of the body produce those oxygen molecules as by-products. Think of them as waste products from all the things that go on in your body, breathing to digestion,' she adds. 'They become toxic when they build up in our cells more than they should.'

Why do they build up? Oh, for any number of reasons: the food you eat, the medicines you take, the air you breathe, the water you drink, from second-hand smoking, even from jet lags. And, yes, if you are overweight, you have more free radicals. Sugary foods are particularly bad, excess sugar in the bloodstream stimulates free radicals. And type 2 diabetes is linked to a rise in free radicals.[1]

In brief, free radicals are like little bullies for your cells. Normally, your body knows how to handle them. Problem starts if you have too many and they get a free hand to damage cells across your blood vessels and organs. The injuries build up over time into slow-burning flames of chronic inflammation. With age, free radicals bring in progressive and adverse changes to the body. Can they be controlled? Nature, meditation and anti-inflammatory diets can reverse the havoc of oxidative stress, says my therapist.

All the Jargon You Need to Know

You will need to pick up a whole lot of medical jargon to understand the state of your health in the new millennium. With ideas and tools coming in from physics, chemistry, computational sciences, mathematics and engineering, the 'new biology' of the twenty-first century goes beyond organs, muscles and tissues and into cells, genes and molecules. And inflammation is at the heart of this science. Inflammation is a word we have all heard, but do we really know what it means?

If you have sprained an ankle, cut a finger or been stung by a bee, you would have experienced inflammation. Pain, redness, swelling, tenderness and heat are the signature symptoms of inflammation in your body. It's the powerful battle your immune system wages to protect and heal you, if the barrier between your body and the world outside is breached, say, by an infection, an injury or an irritant. Because immune cells are present in your whole body—interconnected, interrelated and interdependent—inflammation can manifest as a range of diseases.

Is this the same as chronic inflammation? Not really. For that, you need to understand how your immune system works: first, the frontline of your immune system consists of white blood cells that patrol your body. Then, there are the macrophages in the tissues that can surround, kill and digest invading pathogens, debris and dying cells.[2] When macrophages call for support, wave after wave of immune cells arrive. Uncontrolled, they can cause serious harm both to the invaders as well as to your healthy tissues. A last wave of chemicals is released, then quickly the process subsides and healing begins. This is basic inflammation—transient and beneficial in nature.

Problem arises when the immune system refuses to shut down—perhaps because the pathogen persists, or foreign bodies cannot be broken down, or there is extensive damage to healthy tissue—and becomes uncontrolled. By mistake, it turns on itself and attacks the body. The longer this goes on, the more the chances of inflammation becoming chronic: like a slow-burning fire, smouldering and simmering for months and years.[3] Chronic inflammation has many features of acute inflammation but is usually of low grade and persistent, resulting in tissue degeneration. This then triggers some of the most challenging diseases of our time: from diabetes, heart disease, Alzheimer's, cancers, arthritis, asthma, gout, psoriasis, anaemia, Parkinson's disease and multiple sclerosis to depression, among others.

The Science of Eating

Chronic inflammation interferes with the most important function of your body: metabolism, that is, all the chemical reactions by which what you eat and drink is converted into energy. Metabolism provides energy for movement and physical exertion as well as all for all the invisible functions when you are at rest: thinking, breathing, blood circulation, adjusting hormone levels, repairing cells and so on. With chronic inflammation, metabolism gets deranged. And you get a cluster of abnormalities:

high blood sugar, increased blood pressure, excess body fat around the waist and abnormal cholesterol levels. Together they are called metabolic syndrome.[4]

If you have ever thought about your diet and health, about type 2 diabetes, weight management or heart disease, you must have noticed how doctors and scientists pepper conversations with catch phrases and jargon that are foreign to the uninitiated. Even nine out of 10 sufferers of these diseases will not be able to say what these terms mean or why they matter to them. Here is a simplified way of looking at few such obscure terms on metabolism and inflammation.

Do you know what 'good' carbs and 'bad' carbs are? When you eat carbohydrates, they are broken down into simple sugars. Bad carbs digest fast and boost your blood sugar levels quickly. Examples are cooked potato, white bread, bananas, pasta, white rice, candies, chocolates and chips. Then, there are the 'good' carbs that digest more slowly and raise blood sugar gradually. Examples are starchy foods, and sugars you find in fruits and dietary fibres.

In the past two decades, with dieting and weight-loss obsessions sweeping the world, public interest in all things glycaemic (the word comes from 'glucose') has exploded. From popular diet books to magazine articles, television advertisements to talk shows, social media to sport nutrition platforms, great claims are being made about low glycaemic diets—from losing extra weight and controlling chronic diseases like diabetes to optimizing health and well-being. So what exactly are these?

When we eat, digestible carbs are absorbed from

the intestine into the bloodstream. As blood sugar rises, the hormone insulin is released from the pancreas and causes blood sugar to fall to normal levels in a short time. The magnitude of this rise and fall in blood sugar, and the duration over which it occurs, are called glycaemic response (GR). It varies for different carbs, the amount of food consumed, the extent of cooking, the ripeness of food, the amount of fat or protein in the food and so on. Of the tools that help measure GR, the most significant are glycaemic index (GI) and glycaemic load (GL).

GI is a ranking of carbohydrate-containing foods on a scale of zero to 100, with pure glucose at the top and other carbs getting a number commensurate with its effect on blood sugar levels. Sweet corn (GI 55), for instance, raises blood glucose levels 55 per cent as much as pure glucose. Foods that are below 55 are termed 'low GI foods', foods in the range of 55–70 are mid-GI and those with over 70 are considered high GI foods. Cooking or processing can raise GI. For instance, raw carrots have a GI of 16, while for cooked carrots it is 92. Ripeness and storage time also affect GI.

The problem is, GI applies only when food is consumed on an empty stomach. What's more, GI does not take into account the amount of food consumed. It is determined by a serving containing 50 grams of carbohydrate, minus the fibre. But something like beets, for instance, has a GI of 64, but just 13 grams of carbs per cup. One would need to consume nearly four cups of beets to cause that spike in blood sugar levels. So, GL has emerged as an alternative. It accounts for the amount of carbohydrate per serving. Lower GI and GL diets, which do not cause blood sugar levels to spike, have been found to reduce inflammation.

The Case against Western Diet

What sets metabolism aflame? The 'elephant in the room', seems to be the way we eat now, or the 'Western diet'.[5] With the globalization of taste, foods high in fat and sugar—processed foods, fast foods, convenience foods and sugary soft drinks—have spread to both sides of the global village as the 'modern diet' of our times.[6] With spiralling rates of lifestyle diseases becoming a public health concern of global epidemic proportions, the Western diet is being blamed as a cause for chronic metabolic inflammation, or metaflammation.[7]

These are foods that our caveman ancestors would not have known: namely, refined cereals, refined sugar, saturated fats, trans-fats, fatty meats, and foods with added salt and sugar. They also would not have consumed sugar in such significant amounts.[8] In a review of sugar consumption in 18 developed countries, it has been found that total sugar intake as a percentage of energy ranges between 13.5–24.6 per cent in adults—much higher than the recommend free sugars intake of 5–10 per cent daily by the WHO.[9]

Check out some of the common nutrients of Western diet: meat, butter and cheese, for instance, contain saturated fatty acids that can raise 'bad' cholesterol LDL in blood. Sugars and refined grains can promote weight gain and disturb the balance in our gut microbiome. Red meat and other animal products, when taken in excess, can increase amino acids purine, carnitine and histidine in blood, leading to a range of inflammatory diseases: from gout and heart disease to diabetes.

According to scientists, the transition from Paleolithic nutrition to Western diets, without corresponding genetic adaptations, have disrupted the finely tuned human metabolism that evolved over millions of years. Overconsumption of foods that are poor in natural antioxidants, fibres, vitamins and minerals tip our immune system into producing excessive amounts of cells that can cause damaging inflammation.[10] Energy-dense and calorie-rich Western diet is marked by high GL, high oxidative stress and high levels of free radicals, provoking rapid rise in blood sugar and weight gain.

Mother of All Inflammations

Think of the earliest female figurines known to us: the Three Mothers. The tiny statuettes unearthed at excavation sites in Europe have been named Venus of Hohle Fels, Venus of Dolní Věstonice and Venus of Willendorf. Short, squat, broad-shouldered and abundantly endowed, with overhanging stomach and obtrusive genitalia, they have been dated 40,000–25,000 years ago. Were they aspirational symbols of femininity and fashion, like the Barbie dolls of our time? To modern endocrinologists, however, they are icons of obesity and metabolic syndrome.[11] Chronic inflammation may have been the bridge connecting them.

For long, scientists have considered fat to be inert, just a storehouse of fuel in the form of triglycerides. The new science of obesity shows that fat—especially the white fat that wraps around abdominal organs deep inside your body—is active. Unlike fat in other parts of the body, visceral fat produces a variety of chemicals that can cause chronic inflammation. Take, for instance, macrophages that rise exponentially in fat tissue during obesity. There is also the cytokine molecule, which is released in excess in obesity, leading to inflammation.

A typical example is the hormone leptin. High leptin levels make people feel full and they stop eating. With high-sugar, high-fat diets, however, the body stops responding to leptin. In people with obesity, leptin levels are unusually high, yet they continue to be hungry, which promotes overeating. This makes fat cells produce even more leptin, triggering cytokines and setting off inflammation. Cytokines also block insulin. As a result, sugar levels rise in the blood and more calories are stored as fat—a path to diabetes.

As obesity progresses, fat cells grow larger and larger. Unable to store fuel any more, they start spitting out molecules into the bloodstream. That triggers chronic low-grade inflammation. The greater the presence of visceral body fat, the higher your risk of contracting serious medical conditions. Obesity and diabetes increase oxidative stress, making it difficult for oxygen to reach where it should. The risk of developing heart failure becomes higher in this setting.

This might be a moment to think about our three obese mothers of yore: did they become fat on high-sugar and high-fat diets, although food was generally scarce? Were they high-status women who could eat to excess? Were they born with genes that made their immune systems overreact to their environment and secrete cytokine-like molecules? Did they have hyperactive immune systems, insulin resistance, diabetes and heart disease? One may never know, but this is certain: at a time when people died randomly of infection, injury, starvation or childbirth, the layers of fat on the Three Mothers made them well suited for survival. In this age of calorie-dense, nutrient-poor junk and fast foods, they would surely have died young.

Breathing Dirty Air

Billions of tiny toxic particles are swirling around you. Nasty little molecules of black-and-brown carbon, dust and dirt, sand and smoke, minerals and salts, volatile compounds and ozone, pollens and spores. They cloak your city in a semi-transparent haze, layer the sky with unholy orange clouds and hug the ground in suspended animation. The smallest of the small flecks, thousands of which can fit into a full stop in a sentence, sneak past the flypaper-like mucus of your nose and throat. They travel deep into your body and attack its ability to process sugar.

The villain at work is the tiniest form of particulate matter: PM 2.5, a noxious mix of solid fragments and liquid droplets suspended in air. At 2.5 microns in size and rich with a great variety of toxic metals, they put severe pressure on your pancreas, which can't pump out insulin. Without insulin, your blood gets heavy with sugar, but your cells are starved of it. For survival, your body starts burning proteins, fats and muscles to generate energy.

What you face in the process is inflammation.

The effect of ambient air pollution on a constellation of health complications linked to sugar pathways and mechanisms is getting increasing attention. Scientists have tried to understand for long what exactly causes diabetes, how it happens and why some people are at a higher risk. Poor diet, lack of physical activity, family history, excessive weight and age have been blamed so far. A host of new global studies are pointing to an additional surprising culprit: air pollution.

Air pollution causes more than nine million deaths from stroke, heart disease, lung cancer and chronic respiratory diseases per year.[12] For the first time, air pollution is being linked to cardiometabolic diseases, combining a derangement of both the heart and metabolic systems. Recognized as a disease entity by the WHO, people with cardiometabolic diseases are twice as likely to suffer fatal heart disease or stroke as those who do not have it.[13] These diseases are also rising at a faster clip in countries undergoing rapid economic transformation, like India.

Particulate matters are emitted by various industries, by air contaminants that react in the atmosphere, by vehicles, airplanes, trains and ships. Scientists are beginning to understand what makes PM 2.5 so harmful: even if you cough or sneeze, it is very difficult to expel it out of your body, thus making it dangerous. New research shows how inflammation induced by these lethal air particles leads to diabetes.[14] Air pollution is likely to cause 3.2 million new cases of type 2 diabetes every year globally.[15]

Researchers are probing the biological mechanisms

behind diabetes caused by air pollution. It has been found that PM 2.5 also attacks the liver, which possesses the remarkable ability to store, produce and keep blood sugar levels steady. During a meal, the liver stores sugar for a later time, when your body needs it—for instance, between meals or overnight. PM 2.5 blocks sugar intake in the liver, and causes oxidative stress and inflammation, leading to abnormality in sugar regulation.[16]

Health effects of air pollution on inflammation and diabetes have been scarcely studied in developing countries. Studies on air pollution in China have found that long-term exposure to air pollution can increase the risk of diabetes.[17] The study indicates that exposure to a range of particulate pollution—PM 1, PM 2.5, PM 10, SO2, NO2 and O3—might adversely affect the risk of developing diabetes.[18] Given the coexistence of high air pollution and an epidemic of diabetes in China, the results are of significance to public health policymakers.

Tale of Two Chemistries

Let's talk about two networks that are understood little, and thus, sadly undervalued, when it comes to sugar. One is the vagus nerve, the longest nerve bundle in your body, which spreads all the way from your brain to your colon—like a vagabond without direction or destination. The other is cortisol, the fascinating hormone that gets a bad rap for priming you for a 'fight or flight' response when under stress and is blamed for everything from weight gain to stroke.

As more and more scientists try to pin down their

exact mechanism, new research reveals that both may be the missing links in chronic inflammation and both have a stake in sugar. In 2020, two groups of scientists identified for the first time how the vagus pathways drive sugar cravings.[19] Yet another study has shown the detrimental role of cortisol in high blood sugar levels of people with diabetes.[20]

When the brain perceives physical or psychological stress, it starts pumping powerful hormones such as cortisol from the adrenal glands above the kidneys. Instantly, the heart beats faster, blood pumps harder, blood pressure shoots up, sugar rises in the blood and the senses get sharper. And we are ready to act: fight or flight. Once the situation is resolved, everything returns to normal. Research shows that moderate amounts of stress is actually good for us.[21] It can improve our memory, heart function and resistance to infection.

What if the stressors do not go away or new ones arise repeatedly? Our body keeps pumping out cortisol, which floods our system with sugar, setting up inflammation. This, in turn, keeps cortisol levels soaring. Over time, a range of diseases develops: indigestion, insomnia, obesity, chronic fatigue, thyroid disorders, dementia, depression and diabetes to heart attack. It also leads to lowering of life expectancy. At a time when we work too hard, feel overwhelmed by the toxic challenges of modern life and have few ways of managing our stress, excessive cortisol becomes a roller coaster that ultimately takes us straight down.

The role of the vagus nerve holds immense promise in this setting. The pathway of vagus is like a super information highway between the brain and the body. With its vast network of nerves, stationed like spies around our internal organs, the vagus nerve is like a walkie-talkie that keeps updating the brain on what's going on inside the body via electric impulses. It also controls innumerable jobs: from resting, digestion, breathing, sweating, talking and controlling heart rates to modulating blood sugar levels.

When the vagus nerve gets wind of an impending inflammation, say, the presence of cytokines, it alerts the brain and draws out chemicals that can calm the immune system. When the primary stress hormone cortisol keeps rising, the vagus nerve tells your body to wind down by releasing the chemical messenger acetylcholine, which dilates blood vessels, increases bodily secretions and slows down heart rate. With its wide reach, the vagus nerve sends instructions across the body to release enzymes and proteins such as prolactin, vasopressin and oxytocin, which regulate anxiety, sociality and the ability to cope with stress.

People with a stronger vagal tone (or how strong your vagus nerve is) are likely to recover faster from stress, injury or illness. The anti-inflammation function of the vagus nerve has made it an attractive therapeutic target connected to inflammation, immune system regulation and metabolism.[22] Both implantable and non-invasive vagus nerve stimulators have been approved in Europe and the US to treat epilepsy, depression, pain and cluster headaches that occur in cyclical patterns. Growing evidence suggests similar stimulation for stress response, chronic inflammation, as well as mood and anxiety disorders.

Are You Inflammaging?

Just in case you did not know, there is a new term on the block: 'inflammaging'. Decoded, it is the chronic low-grade inflammation that develops as you age. From an evolutionary perspective, it's a trail of damage marked by years: the toll taken on your body by malicious pathogens, damaged cells, debris of dead cells, misfolded proteins, misplaced molecules, an overreaction here, a delayed response there, excess nutrients and footprints of changing gut microbiota. That makes chronic diseases the result of 'inflammaging'.[23]

One of the most exciting discoveries of recent times, which won the 2009 Nobel Prize in Physiology or Medicine, is telomeres.[24] Telomeres are the protective cap on the tips of your chromosomes which carry your genetic material. That means your chronological age and biological age are not always the same. Chronological age measures the number of years that has passed since your birth to the given date. Biological age measures the length of your telomeres, because they get shorter with age. Going by that, scientists can now see how fast you are ageing and your life expectancy. Short telomeres are linked not just to premature ageing but also to several diseases, especially cancers. Scientists still haven't completely come to understand what causes telomeres to get shorter, but chronic low-grade inflammation has now been linked to it.

The incontrovertible truth of the biology of ageing is this: immune defenses decline with age. For instance, your Natural Killer Cells, a major immunological weapon, become less effective at destroying cells infected with a virus, as you age. At the same time, inflammation in tissues throughout your body goes up with age. Even a perfectly healthy 60-year-old will have higher levels of immune cells like cytokines involved in inflammation than younger people. Add to it fat tissues, which increase inflammation and render overweight people more vulnerable to ageing and diseases. There are also more cells that stop dividing with age and secrete substances like cytokines. In fact, the greater the number of inflammatory factors, the steeper the cognitive decline, especially memory loss.

Well-Being and Inflammation

Can inflammaging be controlled? I mull over that question at the health retreat as I watch hundreds of butterflies fluttering into a blue sky, the riot of colours from flowers draped over every nook and niche, the palm trees with glossy leaves casting green shadows, rafts of ducks floating lazily by. As a sense of well-being envelops me, I join the dots.

Ancient healing traditions, from Ayurveda to traditional Chinese medicine, have long advocated the importance of nature to well-being. It's only in the last few decades that science has woken up to the new wave of interest in the interdependence of health and nature. Living close to nature and spending time in green spaces has significant and wide-ranging health benefits, reports new research.

With data collected from 20 countries, scientists have measured how exposure to green spaces reduces the risk of type 2 diabetes, improves heart rate, blood pressure, stress and cortisol levels.[25] People living near green spaces have more opportunities for physical activity, while diverse bacteria present in natural ecosystems benefit their immune system and reduce inflammation.

Elsewhere, scientists are reviewing data on pro- and anti-inflammatory foods, engaging in debates over what makes a wholesome diet, conducting studies on the health benefits of diets rich in fibres and polyphenols (chemicals that protect against oxidative stress and are abundant in plants), probing the links between diet and gut microbiome and designing diets as a therapeutic tool for disorders with an inflammatory basis.

Exciting possibilities are opening up as scientists try to reboot the vagus nerve as a brake on stress response. This nerve seems to control breathing and gets activated by deep breathing. Scientists are exploring if meditation and yoga can stimulate it. It is well known that in both these forms, the body releases feel-good, anti-anxiety, longevity, anti-ageing and sleep molecules, while the stress hormone cortisol calms down. The vibration you experience on chanting, say, 'Om', seems to activate this nerve through its branches in your ears.[26] The vagus nerve is stimulated by the vocal cord. So sing, hum and laugh as much as you can. They will lift your mood, boost your immune system and flood your body with happy molecules.

7

The Great Nutrition Transition

Jhingru Bhuiyan died on a July morning of 2018. Shrunken and grey, he looked much older than his 42 years. His children, Chandan, five, and Gunja, just seven months old, clung to their mother, Rubi Devi, as the word spread about yet another starvation death. Newspapers flashed headlines and police officers asked probing questions: when had he eaten last? What and how much? In the end, Jhingru's body was lifted from the funeral pyre for an autopsy. The state needed to figure out if it was really death by starvation or was his family cadging for sarkari largesse.

That was also a week of mourning for the nation. India's most ambitious mission to the moon, Chandrayaan 2, scheduled to take off on its voyage of 3.84 lakh kilometres at a whopping $141 million, had missed its tryst with destiny due to technical snags. Jhingru unfortunately never had a date with destiny when he was alive. He lived at the edge of an obscure village called Dondagada, in Jharkhand, eking out a living somehow, until struck by stroke and paralysis in the last year of his life. While his life went by in oblivion, in death, he received some attention. What made his death headline worthy was the claim made by his wife that they had not eaten for 10 days before his death because she could not procure food grains.

I caught up with endocrinologist Dr Ambrish Mithal.[1] He had monitored anti-corruption activist Anna Hazare's metabolic parameters during his famous hunger strike at Jantar Mantar, Delhi, in 2011.[2] How long can one go without food? He explained that a well-nourished, 70-kilogram man would have fuel reserves for about one to two months, but carbohydrate reserves are depleted in a day. In just three to five days, fasting can become dangerous, as the body starts breaking down the liver. This is indicated by rising blood ketone—substances produced by the liver when the body doesn't have enough glucose to use as an energy source. People with excess body fat, however, can last 12–24 weeks.

If you think hunger is in the stomach, think again. It's the brain that signals the body's need for food. And your brain is expensive: more than any other organ in your body, it is the brain that needs energy. Sugar is its primary food. A starving body starts breaking down its stored sugar: first in the fat cells, then in the liver. Toxic by-products—ketone bodies—are produced in the liver within weeks as fuel for the brain, although their rising levels can be lethal. Then, the sugar stored in the muscles is attacked. Weakness, disorientation and low immunity precede the final collapse of the body.

Awe and admiration for self-fasting heroes go back a long time in our history: Mahatma Gandhi, a frail man with an iron will, never went beyond 21 days in any of his 15 fasts; freedom fighter Jatindra Nath Das fasted for 63 days at Lahore jail in 1929 and succumbed to it; Chipko leader Sunderlal Bahuguna could withstand 74 days in 1997. In recent times, yoga guru Ramdev's fast petered out after nine days in 2011; it was 11 days of fast-unto-death for K. Chandrasekhar Rao, who won his demand for a separate Telangana state in 2009; the same year, Dravida Munnetra Kazhagam (DMK) supremo late M. Karunanidhi's fast for Sri Lankan Tamils had ended in half a day.

What happens when you are forced to starve? Memories of people begging for rice water during the Bengal famine of 1943, when over three million people died of hunger, still linger in family lore and literature. In September 2017, when Santoshi Kumari, 11, of Simdega district in Jharkhand, died, her last words to her mother, 'rice, rice', left a scar on the nation's psyche.[3] The Right to Food Campaign reports at least 56 starvation deaths in the last five years, mainly in Jharkhand, Uttar Pradesh, Odisha, Bihar, Chhattisgarh, Karnataka, Delhi, West Bengal and Maharashtra. Jhingru and Santoshi are but faces in that gallery of the dead.

Pangs of Hidden Hunger

There was not an inch of room in Albert Ekka Chowk, at the heart of Ranchi. A hotspot of political rallies, it was overflowing with protestors of all types: activists, students, farmers and tribals. Some were holding bows and arrows, others beating drums. They were all raising slogans on different issues at the same time via multiple public announcement systems. Somewhere there was economist Jean Drèze and his fellow Right to Food activists. Was Jhingru in their list of starvation deaths? Did they know where Dondagada was?

The road from Ranchi meanders through a mysterious landscape of rich red earth and ancient rocks, undulating hills and mossy trickles, towering trees and green voids, glorious networks of rivers and waterfalls. Dondagada, however, is in the back of beyond. Google Maps give it a miss, signals fall silent and local people misguide visitors when asked for directions. Balram, a Right to Food activist and Supreme Court-appointed adviser to the state, who once worked closely with Gandhian socialist leader, Jayaprakash Narayan's movement in Bihar, knows the area by instinct. Guided by him, we finally reach gram Dondagada, district Chatra, block Kanhachatti, and panchayat Jamri Bakaspura.

Visitors for Rubi? The whole village comes calling and everybody wants to cram into that little thatched hut with polished mud floor at the edge of the village. Away from the crowd, she says, she has been begging for food from her neighbours ever since Jhingru became ill a year ago. They have a little bit of land, but with Jhingru unwell, it has been lying fallow. What about their ration cards? They have been struck off the list, she explains, because the Aadhaar linking failed and the ration shop owner refused to relent despite repeated requests. The family has been living on rice and only rice for the past several months. The last 10 days before his death, there was not a single grain of rice at home and the *chullah* (hearth) had grown cold.

Does her son go to school? No, not regularly. He has had to stay at home to help take care of his ailing father. Had he gone to school, he would have got hot lunch with eggs, under the midday meal programme. 'Surely that would have helped?' we ask. Eggs are given only twice a week, she says, and it's just one meal a day. That's why he has stayed at home, so that she could go out and procure food. 'He is not the only one, many of the village children don't go to school. They help their parents on the field or with housework, so that everyone gets food at home,' she says.

At the local school, barefoot children in outsized uniforms eagerly wait for the visitors. On talking to them, we find out what they had eaten through the day: sabzi with roti mostly, some with rice. Only one girl says she has had milk that morning. Do they like eggs? 'Yes,' they shout uproariously. How about fruits? 'Yes,' they roar again. Do they have fruits every day? Silence. The girl, who had milk, raises her hand: 'I had a mango yesterday. We have a tree.' The teacher shows us a height and weight chart that the school maintains: none of the students have reached their ideal height or weight.

Are the children growing up well? Without wholesome foods like milk and fruits, they are likely to grow up with a different type of hunger that is invisible—called 'hidden hunger'—which robs children of vitality at every stage of life. Even if stomachs are full, missing vital vitamins and minerals—such as iodine, iron, folate, selenium, vitamin A and zinc—give children short stature for their age (stunting) and low weight for height (wasting). And

India tops the world in having children who don't just go to bed hungry but are stunted, wasted and underweight from 'hidden hunger'.[4]

While 'hidden hunger' may remain hidden in plain sight, children carry this burden for the rest of their lives, battling chronic tiredness, low immunity, infections, aches and pains, anxiety, ulcers, restlessness, irritability, depression, brain fog, night blindness and goitre. Poor intake of folate and B vitamins have been linked to increased risk of stroke (was Jhingru's stroke and paralysis triggered by malnutrition?).[5] There is growing evidence that nutritional deprivation in childhood and 'hidden hunger' increase the risk of numerous chronic diseases later in life by raising blood sugar levels higher than normal.[6]

Stunting and wasting, in particular, are linked to underdeveloped brain and long-lasting harmful consequences: from diminished mental ability and learning capacity, to poor school performance and reduced earnings, along with increased risks of nutrition-related diseases such as diabetes, hypertension, obesity, kidney and heart diseases. It is likely that Jhingru faced hunger, not just for those 10 days before his death, but his whole life. Can the children of his village meet their full physical and intellectual potential in the face of such malnutrition?

'The State shall regard raising the level of nutrition and standard of living of its people and the improvement in public health as among its primary duties,' states Article 47 of the Constitution of India. After 75 years of Independence, however, alarming statistics do the rounds: one-third of the world's malnourished live in India; one-third Indians do not have enough food to eat; one-third of India consumes unhealthy diet.[7] India is among the worst performers on the hunger front, ranking below China, Nepal, Myanmar, Bangladesh and Sri Lanka in the Global Hunger Index.[8]

Side by side with stick-thin hunger, diabetes stalks the countryside. The underpinnings of undernutrition and diabetes have now started to emerge. It seems that underweight people with diabetes have higher levels of HbA1c sugar (the amount of sugar attached to haemoglobin in blood) as well as higher levels of the hormone insulin. The troubling finding is that they develop an imbalance in the immune system; it dampens down the protective immune cells, leaving them vulnerable to infections and diseases of inflammation: diabetes, heart disease, stroke, cancers or dementia.

Surprised by Diabetes in Village India

In 1989, when Chennai-based diabetologist Dr A. Ramachandran decided to study diabetes in rural India, cities were blamed for the alarming curve of the disease in India. Diabetes was seen as a disease of affluence: it happened to people who could afford to overconsume high-calorie, high-fat and high-sugar diets. In the wake of economic reforms in the 1990s, income levels started rising much faster than ever before in India. Couch-potato lifestyle, poor eating habits and persistent stress were becoming visible in city life. By 2001, six major Indian cities showed not just high prevalence of diabetes but also high rates of impaired glucose tolerance (IGT, meaning blood sugar is higher than normal, but not high enough to warrant diabetes).[9]

Dr Ramachandran chose to study a group of predominantly agrarian villages of low-income farmers, with the intention of revisiting them in a few years, to figure out changes with time and economic development. In 2003, however, he had to change his plans. So drastic was the economic change in these villages that their profile had changed completely. They were no longer farmers' villages: with a major automobile industry nearby, most of the young village population was now employed there. He chose three different villages instead, which were identical to the earlier group and had minimum interface with cities and the least migration rate.

What he found was an eye-opener: the prevalence of diabetes had increased three-fold in 14 years, prediabetes was occurring at a younger age and obesity—especially, belly fat—was rising. All this was not happening in a vacuum: by every parameter, their living standards had improved as reflected in the far greater use of electricity (up from 50.6 per cent in 1989 to 95.1 per cent in 2003), water supply (from 68.6 per cent to 96.3 per cent), motorized transport (from 86.6 per cent to 93.4 per cent) and medical facility (from 87.5 per cent to 96.6 per cent).

There was a sea change in the way they lived and worked now. Just 22.8 per cent were engaged in strenuous manual activity in 2003, compared to 80 per cent in 1989. About 48 per cent were engaged in sedentary professions (they also had a significant association with diabetes).

In 2003, women were found to confine themselves to household chores, unlike in 1989, when women were also engaged in manual and field work. This was a direct result of more money in hand: from about ₹254 a month, family incomes had spiralled upward exponentially to ₹1,413 a month. Not surprisingly, there was a 230 per cent rise in watching television at home between 1989 and 2003. All these parameters had led to decreased energy expenditure and greater tendency to put on weight.

As the villagers started earning more, what changed the most was their pattern of eating. In 1989, a typical village meal consisted mainly of cereals, with negligible amounts of proteins and fats. By 2003, rice had become a staple food in place of ragi (finger millets), while fat featured more prominently in their diet. In 1989, just about 57.2 per cent of the villagers had three full meals a day. By 2003, the figure had gone up to 70 per cent. Higher income also brought improved education. In 1989, about 95 per cent of the population had primary school education, but by 2003, over 47 per cent had completed higher secondary education, with 4 per cent securing college or technical degrees. Education had brought awareness about diabetes: over 60 per cent of the people were already being treated for diabetes by the time Dr Ramachandran and his team arrived for field work.

A Passion for White Rice

For Indians, nothing evokes nostalgia more than the sight of snow-white rice at the centre of every meal. The memory of food is precious. The tradition of eating tells us about our roots, our identity and our heritage. The memory of food, however, can also be precarious, evolving and changing with our everyday reality. And sometimes, it is an idealized version of what we remember. Our passion for rice is one such. Indians have traditionally eaten rice, but they have also eaten an abundance of other grains. We have also not eaten white rice until the rice mills arrived in the early twentieth century. Yet, like every memory, this too has enormous capacity to impact the way we eat, live and thrive—or die.

If there is anyone trying to set this wrong right, it is Dr Viswanathan Mohan of Chennai.[10] For the last 40 years, he has been studying the role of the common cereal staple—white rice—behind India's rising diabetes epidemic and trying to improve the Indian diet by replacing white rice with the nutritious whole grain, brown rice. He has repeatedly undertaken novel research to put to test the nutrition quotient of different varieties of rice and processing in his laboratory. His latest study, conducted in collaboration with scientists across the world, confirms his worst fears: the intake of excess white rice is linked to type 2 diabetes.

When Dr Mohan started probing why we like white rice so much, a group discussion with slum dwellers, as also the residents of non-slum areas, of Chennai, elicited a startling response. Someone said, 'We are lovers of rice. Unless someone is sick or has some health problem, we prefer to eat rice.' Someone else said, 'Only if the rice is white in colour will we be satisfied.' Others said that their family members did not relish unmilled rice. Yet others pointed out that buying white rice was a 'prestige issue'. 'People will think poorly of us if we have brown rice instead of white.' And they all agreed that nobody would stop eating white rice unless the government came out with a health warning.[11] All these comments, not surprisingly, came from people who were overweight or had higher blood sugar.

Unfortunately, whole grain rice is highly nutritious but rots easily. To increase the shelf life of rice, mills remove both the bran (the hard, fibre-rich outer layer, whose pigmentation determines the colour of rice) and the germ (the nutrient-rich core of the grain). Bran and germ are rich in protein, fibre, iron and vitamin B and have a healthy ratio of omega-3 to omega-6 fatty acids. With all that removed, what remains is the carbohydrate (starch). In the name of 'white rice' what you get is highly polished, starchy, refined rice, devoid of all nutrients. The white rice is then processed to improve taste and enhance its cooking properties.

Whole grain rice contains the entire grain. In the rice mill, the grain is simply dehusked before it is sent to the market. It is nutritious, and packed with vitamins, minerals, antioxidants, essential amino acids and fibres. It has a low GI (Glycaemic Index or rise in blood sugar level two hours after consuming food) and does not contribute to high GL in the diet (Glycaemic Load or how much the food will raise your blood sugar level after consuming it). The carbs in white rice turn into sugar rapidly. This is one reason why white rice has been associated with a higher risk of type 2 diabetes, obesity, blood pressure and heart disease. White rice also lacks compounds (lignans and phytochemicals), vitamins and minerals, which in the unpolished brown rice confer protection against cell damage, high blood pressure and fat in blood. Brown rice has consistently been found to aid weight loss and help maintain a healthy body weight.

The largest research, confirming the link between white rice intake and the diabetes epidemic, is out now.[12] Conducted in a span of nine-and-a-half years, across 21 countries, and on 132,373 participants, it shows that the largest consumers of white rice are in South Asia, polishing up about 630 grams a day. More than 450 grams per day (one serving of cooked rice being 150 grams) is associated with an increased risk of diabetes. Dr Mohan, who conceived the study in India, sounds out a warning: we are at the highest risk of developing diabetes. Next in line is Southeast Asia (the mean consumption is 239 grams/day). These are followed by China, the Middle East, Europe, Africa, South America and North America.

The modern Indian diet is particularly high in refined carbohydrates—white rice and white wheat—and low in protein, compared with other dietary traditions. The solution is to reduce the proportion of refined carbohydrates in our diet and to include more legumes and pulses (such as Bengal gram, green gram, black gram, rajma/kidney beans, etc.) to enhance the protein and fibre content and reduce the glycaemic load. Along with healthy fats (monounsaturated fats), plenty of green leafy vegetables and some fruits, the Indian diet could become a lot more healthy.

The Nutrition Paradox

Undernutrition and overnutrition are two sides of the same coin: malnutrition. It's a trajectory that spans both the poor and the rich, with each giving a different face to the same statistics: one-third of the world's malnourished live in India; one-third of India do not have enough food to eat; one-third of India has unhealthy diet.[13]

Economists would call the shift—from unrefined sugar to refined sugar—a historical market trend. Public health specialists would sound the alarm on a health disaster in slow motion. Epidemiologists would predict the beginning of a 'nutrition transition', leading towards current and future disease burdens from non-communicable (chronic) diseases: strokes, most heart diseases, most cancers, diabetes, chronic kidney disease, osteoarthritis, osteoporosis, Parkinson's disease, autoimmune diseases, Alzheimer's disease, cataracts and others.

Summed up as a concept, nutrition transition describes the worldwide prevalence of undernutrition and obesity over the last few decades. Coined by Barry M. Popkin, American scholar of nutrition, the theory links economic development as the driver that leads to shifts from diets rich in minimally processed foods of vegetable origin to diets high in meat, fat, sugar and processed foods.[14]

It's a ticking time bomb in a country obsessed with all things sweet, because refined sugar is one of the key nutrients (along with sodium, saturated fats and trans-fats) linked to the changes that lead to nutrition transition: from diets based on traditional grains or starchy roots, locally grown legumes, other vegetables and fruits, and limited foods of animal origin towards more varied diets that include preprocessed food, more foods of animal origin, more added sugar and fat, and often, more alcohol. High-income countries, for instance, have shifted from diets dominated by complex carbohydrates to diets with more fats, added sugar and protein.

Under this concept, with an increase in income, food consumption patterns start changing. It begins with food insecurity, poverty and an increased prevalence of people who are underweight, wasting and stunting. Some segments of this population gain excess weight with socio-economic improvement, although undernutrition persists, especially in rural areas. As people move into cities, their food supplies change dramatically. Urban foods contain more energy from fats, sugar, processed and highly refined cereals than rural diets. With this diet, their food habits and body composition start to change.

At a more advanced stage, there is heavy intake of fatty processed food, added and artificial sugar and meat. While undernutrition drops, the sceptre of obesity and chronic diseases is raised. These factors are worsened by lack of physical activity and leisure, leading to rapid increase in overweight and obesity. The transition is often marked by trade liberalization and reduction of tariffs. Lack of adequate regulations on food safety opens the door to a world of low-quality processed food, resulting in serious health risks.

Legacy of the Green Revolution

A rush of 'izations'—industrialization, mechanization, urbanization, liberalization and, of course, globalization—are blithely used to depict the complex and tortured course of nutrition transition in India. The most significant story, however, is rarely discussed: the Green Revolution of the 1960s, which won American agricultural scientist, Norman E. Borlaug, referred to as the Father of Green Revolution, a Nobel Prize for Peace in 1970.

For India, it altered millennia-old sustainable systems of agriculture and traditional balanced diets, making us prone to life-threatening chronic diseases. Nearly 60 years later, Borlaug's closest Indian collaborator and plant geneticist, M.S. Swaminathan, questioned the very value of the so-called Green Revolution: 'Quite often discoveries may lead to positive results in the beginning and later produce undesirable effects.'[15]

For centuries, India had followed an ecologically optimal model of agriculture.[16] That meant, small plots of organic farming, where tree covers protected the soil from the sun and heavy rains. Crops and vegetation were planted in layers to enrich the soil, stop erosion and circulate rain water. At the same time, crop rotation allowed the soil to retain nutrients. It was a highly effective ecosystem that had evolved over centuries. People grew what they needed, or gathered from the surroundings—plants, herbs, fruits, fish and livestock. The consumption of traditional coarse grains, pulses and millets—rich sources of vegetable protein with balanced amino acid profile—was exceptionally large.

In the 1940s, Borlaug had established himself as a scientist with an international research project on new methods of agriculture in Mexico, funded largely by the Ford Foundation and the Rockefeller Foundation. He successfully bred what came to be known as miracle seeds of dwarf plants that promised double or triple yield. In 1964, the Indian government, under Prime Minister Lal Bahadur Shastri, was facing acute food shortage, after two years of drought. In 1959, the Ford Foundation had already prepared a report for the Ministry of Food and Agriculture: *Report on India's Food Crisis and Steps to Meet it*. The two foundations introduced the new hybrid seeds: Mexican wheat and Filipino rice.

The bioengineered seeds demanded expensive doses of synthetic fertilizers and heavy irrigation to increase crop yield. The wheat and rice seeds needed to be replaced every four to five years to prevent yield decline. Hybrid seeds of maize and sorghum were also introduced at this time. They needed to be replaced every year. The seeds were expensive, and so were the fertilizers, pesticides and pumps to tap into groundwater reserves, which depleted rapidly with these seeds. The most successful and highly distributed were rice, maize and wheat, especially wheat.

While the US's chemical and agribusiness industries grew massively on the back of their patented seeds and herbicides, India averted food crisis. The Green Revolution, however, resulted in low water tables, depleted soil, reduced genetic diversity of seed bank, a heavy use of chemicals and increased vulnerability to pests and weeds.[17] Small peasant farmers found themselves trapped in a cycle of high interest rates, loans, impoverishment, increased debt and selling of land to afford the Green Revolution package. Super farms started replacing family farms, while reports of farmer suicides started trickling in from around this time.

Most importantly, the Green Revolution changed India's age-old food basket, by changing the system of multiple crops of traditional agriculture to monocropping of rice and wheat. Ever since, successive governments focused entirely on wheat and rice, promoting quick adoption of technology, high-yielding grains, intensive farming, the use of chemical fertilizers and price assurance.

India's rich genetic diversity of thousands of indigenous seeds, grains, cereals and plants, some with high nutritive value, started to disappear. Pulses and millets—inexpensive sources of energy and protein so long—were neglected. The shrinking availability of pulses, even with imports, led to a fundamental change in the nation's food intake: a nutrition transition. As production declined and prices shot up, Indians started shifting to eggs, chicken and fish to fulfil their protein requirement. It's called 'Livestock Revolution', a term coined by The International Food Policy Research Institute (IFPRI).

In most developing countries surveyed by the Food and Agriculture Organization of the United Nations (FAO), energy density contained in food has gone up between 1970 and 1999.[18] The daily per capita supply of fats from animal foods in the developed countries has risen by 4 grams and in the developing world by 14 grams over three decades (1969–99). Whole cereal consumption has fallen in the developing countries, from 60 per cent to 54 per cent in 10 years (1989–99). And consumption of sugar has gone up worldwide during this time, the main source of this increase being carbonated soft drinks.

Unfortunately, the movement towards more fats, salt, sugars and refined foods does not represent optimal nutrition. With large multinational corporations seeking new markets, what has taken a century or more in the developed countries has taken just a few decades in the developing world. The globalization of diet and taste is hastened by trade liberalization: for India, the flashpoint has been the economic reforms of 1991.

As the nutrition transition unfolds, and traditional diets are replaced by new diets, the far-reaching public health impact of chronic diseases becomes evident. The FAO projections forecast the same trend, at least, until the 2030s.

8

A Virus That Loves Sugar

A shadow war is underway. A cloud of aerosols covers an unsuspecting human. He doesn't know, but with each breath he is inhaling thousands of virus particles. They wiggle, bounce and ricochet inside his nose and mouth. And they zigzag down his respiratory tree into the deep recesses of his body. Less than a millionth of an inch wide, they appear to be studded with spikes: proteins, really. But if you take a molecular view, they look like billowy blooms of tulip swaying gently on long stems.

As they undulate and swivel, they look for human cells to dock on. Not just any cell, but ones with special doorways smeared with sugar.[1] The virus knows it won't be allowed in unless it looks and feels comfortably familiar and harmless. And it is ready with stealth ammunition: sugar. Luxuriant sugar molecules swirl around the spikes and hide them, like wolves in sheep's clothing. The virus moves closer to human receptor cells and the spikes begin to dance: up, down, up, down.

The camouflage works. Even the powerful soldiers of the immune army, on constant patrol around the body for nasty entities, pass them by without stopping for a closer look. And cell doorways unlock, fooled. Sugars now prop up spikes in ready-to-infect position. The virus breaks in, grabbing a cell like Velcro. Within minutes, it hijacks the resources and creates thousands of replicas of itself. As the progenies burst out, the cell gets snuffed out, its alarm system defanged. The virus advances, rapidly but stealthily: capture by capture, cell by cell. Within hours, virus particles appear in every teaspoon of the human's blood.

Tripping on High Blood Sugar

The immune army wakes up and launches its massive firepower at the super-aggressive SARS-Cov-2, the novel coronavirus that causes Covid-19. Antibodies, Killer T cells, other snipers and sharpshooters of the body's defence system destroy, target, stalk, neutralize and annihilate the aliens. The immune army also orchestrates wound healing and tissue repair. Some infected cells kill themselves to save the human, a common biological process; some cells record enemy patterns to memory for future recall, so that the predator doesn't evade detection and destruction the next time, unless it changes dramatically.

Unfortunately for the immune militia, the human has high blood sugar: in fact, he has diabetes and hence low immunity. The excess sugar in his blood dampens the immune firestorm—like damp Diwali firecrackers that fail to explode. The immune system expects the thin layer of mucous covering the airway of his lungs to do its job: that is, protect and defend the body by clearing up foreign particles. It is, however, dripping with sugar and fails to work. The sugar, in fact, breaks down the main antiviral defences of the lungs, creating the ideal condition for SARS-CoV-2 to escape the immune blaze and infect with greater venom.

As the war becomes intense, the immune system goes full tilt, to keep the human safe. The surfeit of sugar in his blood, however, makes it hyper excitable. In the ensuing frenzy, cytokine molecules, the foot soldiers of the immune army, tip over. Out of control now, they set off a storm of signals and start attacking multiple organs of the human: the heart, lungs and liver. Fluid builds up in the tiny, elastic air sacs of the lungs. Oxygen level drops, the body temperature goes up, blood pressure drops, blood vessels leak, clots form and organs start to shut down. The army ends up hurting the very body it is meant to protect.

It's an ancient war between mankind and pathogens that has turned a new page in modern times. What remains hidden in this combat is the role of sugar. Scientists now report that the entire lifecycle of the new coronavirus is paved with sugar—from the infection process, the appearance of symptoms to the progression of the disease.[2] Post infection, too, the victorious virus messes with the blood sugar regulation of the body, leading to acute inflammation, raising blood sugar levels further.

Our immune army stands betrayed, defanged and vanquished. The damage done by inflammatory cytokines create abnormalities in the blood vessels, puts insulin in disarray, harms the cells of the pancreas that secrete insulin and damages the liver that produces glycogen hormone.³ Without the concerted effort of insulin and glycogen, blood sugar levels become unmanageable. With high viral load, and uncontrolled blood sugar, the human is now on a downward spiral. He finds refuge in a hospital ICU, with severe complications.

A Double-Edged Sword Called Sugar

The terms of engagement of this battle date back to billions of years of evolutionary pressure: survival of the fittest, something viruses are particularly good at. On an unstoppable march since 2019, the novel coronavirus has been a step ahead of us. We may have congratulated ourselves for developing a range of vaccines against Covid-19 at a never-seen-before speed, but the virus too has continued to mutate into new and more infectious strains, to spread and thrive more easily.

A virus is a particularly enigmatic entity. Neither dead nor alive, it lives like a zombie until it finds a host to latch on to. The moment it does, it invades its cells. Since it cannot reproduce, it creates millions of replicas of itself. In this age-old war with viruses, what's new is the science underpinning it. Nearly a century ago, no one had even seen an individual virus: the first electron microscope was discovered only in 1931. Today, scientists have reconstructed the shape of SARS-CoV-2 down to genes, atoms and molecules. And they are learning lessons that could change the way we think about pathogens forever.

What's also changing is the idea of sugar. If you are under the impression that sugar is just sugar, those shiny, sweet granules in your kitchen, think again. Made up of carbon, hydrogen and oxygen atoms, sugar is a vital building block of life. And our cells love sugar. Sugar feeds them and along with oxygen creates the energy they can use. Of the various forms of sugar, glucose is the most important as it's the primary food for the brain. Sugar also provides the language of communication our cells use to 'talk' to each other, called the sugar code.

That's not all: a canopy of sugar coats every cell in fuzzy profusion and plays a key role in every biological process. This sugar coating is like a unique barcode that protects us, first, by priming our immune system to recognize the sugar on pathogens and, then, to mount attack. With the help of sophisticated analytical technology, science is unravelling this enigmatic world of sugar now.

It's not just us: bacteria and viruses have a sweet tooth, too. Many of them seek out the sugar coating on our cells to infect us. Others have evolved the strategy of tricks and camouflage to evade our immune system by masking themselves in sugar or mimicking our sugar coats. The novel coronavirus is not the only virus to depend on sugar to infect our cells. So do the influenza virus, human immunodeficiency virus (HIV), respiratory syncytial virus, hepatitis C virus and a host of others. Scientists, however, believe that sugar plays out in more complex ways in the novel coronavirus. The sugar coating on corona spikes is unusually lavish.[4] Could it be behind the virus's super infectivity? Efforts are on to develop drugs that can snip off some of the sugars on the virus.[5]

Sugar, in fact, is like a double-edged sword. Its

dysfunction plays a vital role in countless afflictions: from diabetes, heart disease, stroke, arthritis and cancers to ageing. High concentrations of sugar can cause serious organ damage, while low concentrations can lead to loss of consciousness and sudden death. People with diabetes seem to have more sugars attached to their cell doorways, making it easy for the novel coronavirus to infect more cells and create greater viral load, higher risk of hospitalization, intensive care admission and fatal consequences. Thanks to Covid-19, everybody now knows the medical word 'comorbidity'.

Comorbidities and the Crisis of Sugar

Just for the record: about 200 million Indians have high blood pressure, 77 million have high blood sugar and 54.5 million have heart disease.[6] These are just the official estimates. In reality, there are many more people who are not aware of their health conditions, ignoring or escaping the radar of survey. All comorbidities, along with ageing and obesity, have thrown up the toughest challenge during the Covid-19 pandemic.

International teams of scientists are fitting together the puzzle pieces, capturing thousands of patient records, joining the dots of massive meta-analyses and making all possible connections by pooling data from peer-reviewed papers. They now know why some people are more severely affected by SARS-CoV-2. The main culprit is high blood sugar. People at risk of severe Covid-19 seem to have some level of blood sugar abnormality. And, they are invariably at higher risk of poor outcome and mortality.[7]

High sugar level in the blood doesn't just determine how severe the disease will be, but it is in fact the fundamental reason why some people are affected more severely by Covid-19 than others. High sugar level allows the virus to evade the immune army in the lungs, gain deeper access, replicate itself better, kill cells faster, overwhelm the already weakened immune system, set cells on fire and throw up a spray of blood clots.

Sugar is also what links all the comorbidities—diabetes, obesity, hypertension and heart disorder. A tight control of sugar levels is essential in the management of Covid-19.[8] Diabetes, the disease of persistent high blood sugar, is a strong risk factor for Covid-19 severity: one in five Covid-19 patients with diabetes have succumbed to the disease, while 50 per cent of hospitalized patients who died from Covid-19, have had diabetes.[9]

Two measures are generally used to determine blood sugar in our body: FPG (fasting plasma glucose), or blood sugar level after a minimum fasting period of eight hours and PPG (postprandial glucose), or blood sugar level an hour or two after meal. High blood sugar is diagnosed when FPG is over 7 mmol/L (millimoles per litre) (or 126 mg/dL [milligrams per decilitre]) and PPG value is more than 11 mmol/L (or 190 mg/dL). There are many people with modestly raised blood sugar, but because there are no symptoms, they are not aware that they have prediabetes and frequent sugar spikes in their blood.

It is not clear why Covid-19 impacts the elderly more, but one of the many changes that occur with ageing is a steady rise in blood sugar levels: FPG, PPG as well as asymptomatic blood sugar. Hypertension, one of the most common chronic conditions found in the general population, is also one of the most frequent comorbidities in Covid-19-related deaths.[10] In patients below 44 years of age, about 35 per cent of the deaths are associated with hypertension, going up to 70 per cent in patients above 75. Hypertension frequently coexists with the other risk factors such as diabetes, overweight and obesity. In fact, a high proportion of Covid-19 patients have been found to have both diabetes and hypertension.

Hypertension has strong ties with high blood sugar levels: first, high sugar in blood is one of the causes of hypertension; people with high blood pressure are found to have higher fasting sugar in blood;[11] about 70 per cent people with hypertension have disturbed sugar levels, which often remains undiagnosed, but progresses with age.[12] What's more, some beta-blockers, the first drugs prescribed in the management of hypertension, have high blood pressure as its common side effect.[13]

Obesity, even a few extra kilos, has been found to be dangerous in Covid-19. Overweight is a condition where the body mass index (BMI) is between 25 and 30, while obesity is indicated when BMI is over 35 and severe obesity when the value exceeds 40. According to the US health protection agency, the Centers for Disease Control and Prevention (CDC): 'Having obesity...and or severe obesity...increases your risk of severe illness from Covid-19... Having overweight, defined as a BMI > 25 kg/m^2 but less than 30 kg/m^2 might increase your risk of severe illness from Covid-19.'[14] High blood sugar is common in people even with mild obesity.

What often remains unspoken is the risk of high

blood sugar among critically ill patients in hospital ICUs. Called 'stress hyperglycaemia' (also called stress diabetes or diabetes of injury), high blood sugar has been noted even in patients who do not have a history of diabetes due to the stress of coping with disease, hospitalization, and feeding via intravenous lines or feeding tubes. Common drugs used for the treatment of severe viral infection can trigger high blood sugar, too.

In Search of All the Answers

As scientists chip away at data and details, it becomes clear that the link between coronavirus and blood sugar is more complex than imagined. A case in point is the global CoviDiab Registry, set up in June 2020 by an international group of diabetes researchers to probe Covid-19 case reports of people with abnormal blood sugar.[15] Doctors around the world have been uploading anonymous data of patients ever since. The emerging evidence suggests a bidirectional relationship: you can get a severe case of Covid-19 if you have uncontrolled blood sugar and you can get the worst case of abnormal blood sugar if you are Covid-19 positive.

A large-scale Indian study addresses the debate from a different perspective.[16] The researchers focus on psychosocial stress: fear of contracting the virus, of losing loved ones to the disease, of losing one's job and livelihood, enforced lifestyles, the inability to move in open spaces, unavailability of healthy food and difficulty in accessing medical support. Stress manifests in harmful ways: binge eating and reduced physical activity to hormonal imbalance and development of chronic low-grade inflammation. While high blood sugar may eventually get resolved with the amelioration of stress for many, it may persist and get worse for others.

Studies from North India have shown how during the first 45 days of lockdown, carbohydrate consumption and frequency of snacking went up in over 20 per cent people with high blood sugar, exercise duration came down in 42 per cent and weight gain occurred in 19 per cent, while mental stress was reported by 87 per cent.[17] Similar patterns have been reported from across India and in other countries. It is also possible that many people already had undiagnosed diabetes that rapidly progressed during the pandemic. Yet another explanation for higher blood sugar can be delayed diagnosis, due to difficulty (or fear) in accessing lab facilities for blood testing.

The biggest fear at the intersection of sugar and Covid-19 is the emergence of the lethal black fungus (clinically, Covid-19-associated mucormycosis or CAM) that infects the skin, nose, jaw, intestines, lungs and brain of Covid-19 patients, leading to fatal outcomes. Mucormycosis is a serious infection caused by a group of moulds that commonly occurs from fungal spores. India has always recorded the highest prevalence of mucormycosis. Experts blame it on poorly controlled blood sugar as well as the hot and humid environment. A study conducted by AIIMS, Delhi, reports that even in CAM, over 95 per cent cases are associated with high blood sugar.[18]

In the latest round-up of scientific studies on the

sugar–Covid-19 link, the spotlight is on a not-so-well-recognized concept: the gut microbiome, or the trillions of microbes (thousands of species of bacteria, viruses, protozoa, fungi and their genetic material) in the gut, which have co-evolved with humans over millennia and play an important role in sickness and health. In the last decade, scientists have noted that the gut environment can be a vital clue in most serious diseases. The gut profiles of Covid-19 patients are being linked to a more severe disease course. And sugar, once again, seems to play a key role in this puzzle.

Mystery of Sugar in the Covid Gut

There is a jungle inside you. Here, preys, predators and parasites live in a messy balance within the organic sludge of your digestive tract. Hundreds of trillions of bacteria, viruses and fungi float, saunter, scurry and slither along the lining of your food pipe. And they screech, burble and whoosh a million times fainter than the human ear can hear, as they forage, hunt, jostle and compete for survival in that dark terrain. Comprising almost 2 kilogram of your weight, this jungle is your gut microbiome.

Like your fingerprint, your microbiome is unique to you, determined by your genes, gender, age, diet, personal hygiene, the level of activity, the environment you live in and even your life experiences. Scientists call it your invisible organ: the microbes get nourishment from you and in turn supply nutrients to your cells, protect your gut, train your immune system, help digest food, manufacture vitamins, break down toxins and medications, fight invasive pathogens and send messages to your brain via the long vagus nerve about all that is going on in the gut.[19]

Usually, the microbes live in some sort of harmony with you, but not all of them are friendly. Some are neutral, some hostile and some, opportunistic. If your gut microbiome gets disturbed, the negative microbes destroy the richness and diversity of your microbiome by depleting the good ones. An off-balance gut can make you sick by giving you digestive disorders, seasonal allergies, rheumatoid arthritis, psoriasis, chronic fatigue, pain, depression and food allergies. How does the gut microbiome get disturbed? The causes could be many: for instance, when you take medicines; when toxic chemicals enter your body via food; when you consume lots of processed, refined and added sugar; or when you get an infection.

Take, for instance, the little bug, Firmicutes, one of the most abundant types of bacterial flora in your gut. Firmicutes love sugar and simple carbohydrates. It tricks the brain to crave sugars and then generates inflammation, killing off surrounding microbes and feeding on their sugar store. Firmicutes are the 'bad guys', responsible for a range of diseases: obesity, diabetes and allergic asthma to dermatitis. Now, consider Bifidobacteria, a very beneficial bacteria which prevents infections and tumours, lowers cholesterol and boosts brain health. What if Firmicutes count goes up and the count of Bifidobacteria comes down in your gut? A high-sugar diet, so common now, changes the composition and diversity of your gut microbiome, pushing up Firmicutes count and putting your system out of balance.

When bacteria do not live in mutual accord and the 'good' bacteria do not successfully control the 'bad' ones (a process called dysbiosis), it can destroy the balance of your gut microbiome and really harm you. How? Consider your intestine: it helps food nutrients get absorbed in your bloodstream, but it also acts as a barrier, so that food and microbes can't get into your circulation. If this wall gets injured, unwanted gaps may appear. Alien, toxic substances, which are not supposed to get into your bloodstream, leach out. The immune system fires up in self-defence, leading to inflammation and ailments: arthritis, allergies, obesity, type 2 diabetes, fatty liver, heart problems, Alzheimer's and cancer, to name a few. A permeable gut lining has a terrible-sounding medical name: the leaky gut.

In the wake of coronavirus, new research shows that the gut microbiome plays a key role in the severity of Covid-19. The gut microbiome is the weakest in the elderly, the immune-compromised and those with comorbidity—people who fare poorly in combating Covid-19. It is surmised that they develop the leaky gut, allowing the SARS-CoV-2 virus to leach out into the blood stream and spread. It is worth noting that the gut houses 70 per cent of the body's immune cells. This triggers a runaway release of inflammatory chemicals by the immune system, often more deadly than the virus itself. The speculation is not baseless: the gut microbiome affects lung health and plays a key role in acute respiratory distress syndrome (ARDS), a complication of Covid-19.

It was on 30 January 2020 that a 35-year-old man came

to an urgent-care clinic in Washington, US, with a four-day history of cough and low-grade fever. It was the first case of Covid-19 in the US. His vital signs were largely stable, but on the ninth day of the illness, he reported abdominal discomfort and passed loose stool. Genetic sequencing revealed SARS-CoV-2 genes in his stool specimens. This was the first case that indicated a link between Covid-19 and the gut. Altered gut microbiome, especially from chronic conditions and old age, enhances the risk of a leaky gut.[20]

A range of scientific studies since then has shown that SARS-CoV-2 uses both the lung and the gut microbiome to gain a toehold in the body. It prompts a rise in opportunistic, negative gut bacteria and a drop in the friendly varieties. It also pauperizes the gut microbiome of richness and diversity—an essential precondition for good health. What's more, it provokes the gut microbiome of its victims to go out of balance. A study reported in the journal *Gut* shows how the gut microbiome of people with and without Covid-19 are significantly different.[21]

According to this study, Covid-19 patients have higher numbers of noxious bacteria than people without the infection. For instance, the bacteria *Ruminococcus gnavus* or *R. gnavus* (linked to inflammatory bowel diseases) normally occupies less than 0.1 per cent of a healthy gut, but flourishes during Covid-19. Similarly, *R. torques* (linked to autism, sleep disorders and frailty in the elderly) surges up; same is the case with the bacteria *Bacteroides dorei* or *B. dorei* (linked to chronic kidney disease and autoimmune diabetes). All of these produce potent chemicals that directly induce an inflammatory response from the immune system.

The 'good' bacteria, which can influence the immune system response positively, are woefully low in Covid-19 patients. Notable, for instance are *Bifidobacterium* and *F. prausnitzii*. In patients who have recovered, the number of these beneficial bacteria remains low long after they are cleared of the virus. This is what the researchers call 'Long-haul Covid-19 symptoms', which include fatigue, breathlessness and joint pains.

Microbiome research in the time of Covid-19 is at the tipping point of major breakthroughs. Advances in molecular biology, next-generation gene sequencing, big data and innovative diagnostics are opening up a whole new world of possibilities. As Deepak Chopra, the new-age wellness guru, writes:

> A new way of looking at life itself holds out hope and optimism, because the popular image of deadly viruses assaulting humans like microscopic aliens is incorrect. Microbes are the very basis of life. We interact with them constantly, and much more than 99% of the time life is enhanced.[22]

9

Eating with the Gods

It's a memory: a childhood memory of a black-and-white sketch in my Class 3 history textbook. I remember it vividly. It was the only 'story' that spoke to me, amidst a procession of frozen faces staring up from every page: the 'Bearded Man' of Mohenjo-Daro, Emperor Akbar or King Kanishka of the Kushan Dynasty (who did not even have a head). What is it that the sketch was trying to tell me? Of foods, my favourite foods—milk, rice and sugar—of nourishment and its extreme opposite, starvation, and of a mysterious supernatural figure linking them all: the Buddha.

What does my childhood memory tell me now? It asks me to look deep into the food culture of our ancient civilization, probe the collective wisdom of my forebears, investigate the logic of eating that can be traced back to thousands of years and analyse the food values of not just the Buddha but the pantheon of 33 crore gods and goddesses in Hinduism I have inherited. It asks me to follow the science, but not blindly. If science gives us knowledge, religion gives us meaning. Now is the time to reconcile the two over the way we eat and live.

148 • *Sugar*

But, first, let's look at the story. On a full moon night of *Vaisakha* (April or May), some 2,500 years ago, Siddhartha Gautama sat in meditation under an Ashvattha tree on the bank of river Nairanjana. Six years of severe austerities had left his body skeletal. He had followed the strictest of ascetic diets: one piece each of jujube fruit (ber or kul), sesame seed (til) and husked rice a day.[1] Enfeebled by this slow form of starvation, he decided to fortify himself with nourishing food for the supreme spiritual effort: 'Skin, sinew and bone may dry up as it will; my flesh and blood may dry in my body; but without attaining complete enlightenment shall I not leave this seat.'[2]

In the nearby village of Senanigama—Bakraur in present-day Bihar—there lived Sujata. On this day, she was preparing rice milk to offer to the sacred tree under which Gautama sat meditating. The offering of rice milk was special, for Sujata pastured a thousand cows, well-known for the sweetest and most nutritious milk they produced. When she finished preparing the rice milk, she poured it into a gold dish and proceeded to offer it to the tree. She took Gautama to be the spirit of the tree and said: 'Lord, accept my donation, and go whithersoever it seemeth to you good.'[3]

Gautama accepted the sweet, dense milk rice, the food that restored his health. Then, he bathed and cast the bowl into the river. As it floated upstream, along the middle of the river, he realized his spiritual endeavour would succeed that very day. He returned to the tree—called the Tree of Awakening—and took his seat facing east. In the course of the night, he passed through stages of attaining the ultimate knowledge—of causation and cure of the evil of mortality—until at dawn he became wholly awakened as the Buddha. He looked up and saw the morning star and broke into his famous song of victory: 'The transient fades, my heart is free.'[4]

Years later, I live in a world of food conundrum, as torn as the Buddha, perhaps, between wrong foods and the weakening of the body. Science is sounding the alarm: avoid sugar and avoid bad carbohydrates—the prime source of sugar in our diet. We live in a world where sugar is aplenty. Our hungry brain is hardwired for sugar and we are tempted by constant cues of sugar-laden foods from all sides, triggering hunger more often than is good for us. We have lit the fires of chronic inflammation within us, thanks to sugar and air pollution. Can it be dampened down easily? Can our genes and hormones protect us from lifestyles that are at odds with our biology?

Follow the 'Great Middle Path'

The first teaching the Buddha delivered after his awakening was that of the Middle Path, *Majjhimapaṭipada*. He described the human mind as being a party of screeching, chattering, drunken monkeys, all clamouring for attention—envy and fear being the loudest. He showed his students how to breathe, think, eat, walk, meditate and practise moderation in everything to calm the mind. Moderation was also his approach towards food: eat in the middle way, between overindulgence and unrealistic abstinence. The Buddha encouraged his followers to eat simple food, but very few foods were absolutely prohibited and he refused to make vegetarianism compulsory. Remember, alms were the only way a Buddhist monk could survive.

Yagu, a watery rice gruel, was consumed by the monks before going out for alms every morning (a handful of rice boiled in plenty of water with salt, sometimes with sour milk, curd, fruits, vegetables, and even meat or fish). This was taken with *madhugolaka*, a ball of honey and molasses. The Buddha said, it gives life, beauty, ease, strength and intelligence, checks hunger, keeps off thirst, regulates wind, cleanses the bladder and digests raw remnants of food.[5] The midday meal consisted of rice, meat or fish curry, fresh fruits and leafy vegetables. No solid food was allowed after noon, just fruit juice, sugar water or molasses. The five foods he recommended were: *odana* (boiled rice prepared with ghee, meat and fruit); *sattu* (from baked grains of barley, gram flour, wheat or millets); *kummasa* (a boiled mixture of barley [or rice] and pulses); *maccho* (fish) and *mamsa* (meat).

Millennia later, the Buddha's ideas on food and eating are finding new resonance. The Planetary Health Diet, or the first science-based universal healthy reference diet, designed by over 30 world-leading scientists in 2019, chimes with the Buddhist concept of moderation: embrace plants as a source of protein, cut down red meat and sugar consumption by half, double the intake of healthy foods such as fruits, vegetables, legumes and nuts, above all, approach food in moderation.[6] The global food system is broken and industrial agriculture is destroying the environment, as forests are razed and billions of cattle emit climate-warming methane. To nutritionist and physician Walter Willett of Harvard University, who led the Planetary Health Diet study, 'The world's diets must change dramatically.'

There's more: based on the Buddha's idea of mindfulness (or being fully aware of what is happening within and around you at this moment), new approaches are opening up: from relieving stress to high blood pressure to mental health issues. Mindful eating is now being increasingly advocated and applied, led by the Harvard School of Public Health, as the remedy for fast-paced stressful lives. Mindful eating is not about dieting and starving, but being in tune with one's body, mind and the meal in front, with concentration and without distraction. It is an antidote to eating anytime and overeating, because you are not supposed to eat unless you are actually hungry. Studies show, people are more satisfied and eat less when they eat mindfully and without distractions such as the TV or cell phone.

Even more influential today is the Buddha's idea of time-restricted eating, also called intermittent fasting. Instead of focusing on what or how much to eat, it concentrates on when to eat, i.e the time. Buddha laid down the following monastic rules on eating, which he himself followed: no eating of solid foods at the wrong time (after sundown), and not having food at night (one could have drinks, though), as recorded in the Book of the Discipline, *Vinaya-Pitaka*.[7] We have growing evidence that eating in a six-hour period and fasting for 18 hours can trigger a metabolic switch from glucose-based to ketone-based energy, thus curbing stress levels, increasing longevity and a bringing down incidence of diseases, including cancer and obesity.[8]

Milk, Rice and Sugar

The trinity of milk, rice and sugar marked the life of people in ancient India. Those were the main foods offered to gods as *naivedya* and consumed by devotees as *prasada*. They were needed in everyday rituals and in sustaining temples. Around this trinity revolved the lives of the people who called themselves gods: the Vedic Aryans. Essentially pastoral and agrarian people, their lives were focused around their villages, farms, cattle, nature, gods and elaborate gastronomic values and practices.

One of the most important foods for the Aryans and their gods was payasa (payaas), a dessert of rice and milk, slow-cooked with crystal sugar and fragrant spices. A popular dish of ancient India, it has survived as a historic culinary tradition for over 2,000 years. Surprising, because a lot of the other dairy-based recipes that find mention in early texts have disappeared. Payasa, however, got upgraded as temple food in the Common Era and continues to be so across India. Temples across the country are famous for the payasa they offer to the gods, most being Vishnu temples.

At the Jagannath temple in Odisha, where the *mahaprasad* feeds a staggering one lakh people every day, milk, rice and sugar predominate, with *khiri chaula payasa* taking the pride of place. The pink *paal payasam* of the Ambalappuzha Sree temple of Kerala is prepared from pounded red rice and takes about seven hours of slow cooking. At the Sabarimala Temple of Kerala, millions of cans containing Lord Ayyappa's payasam, made of ghee, are sold during the pilgrim season. The Adi Jagannatha Perumal temple of Tamil Nadu may not be as famous as other temples, but its *Thirupullani payasam*, made with local unrefined sugar (*nattu sarkkarai*), is a part of lore.

Ancient Aryans knew how to ferment milk by adding herbs, fruits and plants as coagulants. *Dadhi* (curd) was not only an offering to the gods, it was also a material for many foods. It was eaten with rice, barley or the enigmatic *soma* juice. A mixture of dadhi with boiled milk was called *samnayya* (literally, putting together); butter globules in liquid after dadhi was diluted and churned was called *prasadjya*.[9] A favourite preparation was *payasya* (not payasa), in which dadhi was added to boiling milk. As heat and lactic acid coagulated the milk protein, curd solids and liquid separated. The former (*amiksa*) were mixed with boiled milk, crystal sugar and fragrant herbs. There were other popular items: *shirkarni*, a version of the modern *shrikhand*, buttermilk with sugared and spiced curd.[10]

Payasa cooked with whole grain rice is nutritious and rich in fibre, antioxidants, proteins (in particular the beneficial amino acid lysine), minerals (magnesium, manganese, phosphorus and selenium) and vitamins (niacin, B6 and E). Whole grain rice is a great source of antioxidants, thanks to beneficial plant compounds called phytochemicals, which protect our cells against oxidative damage and reduce the risk of diseases such as diabetes, heart disease and cancer.[11] With white polished rice and sugar, however, payasa today can cause a sudden sugar overload.

Dadhi is going strong across millennia. New research has found a wellspring of nutritive qualities in fermented foods, and especially in natural yogurt. Microbiologists report that eating foods such as yogurt, kefir, fermented cottage cheese, kimchi and other fermented vegetables, vegetable brine drinks and kombucha tea leads to an increase in overall microbial diversity in the digestive tract, with stronger effects from larger servings.[12] Fermented food can dampen down inflammation triggered by harmful bacteria, strengthen the immune system and reduce the risks of type 2 diabetes, heart attack and some cancers. Just remember to use full-fat (and not low-fat) dairy: they have now been linked to lower risks of diabetes, high blood pressure and the cluster of factors (metabolic syndrome) that heighten the threat of heart disease.

In a country ravaged by diabetes, does the Aryan legacy of milk-rice-sugar have any future? I am reminded of the stories of the presidential kitchen during the time of the twelfth president of India (2007–12), Pratibha Patil, who had diabetes but enjoyed her food, and how the chefs at Rashtrapati Bhavan used to come up with innovative recipes. For instance, chef M. Ramachandra Iyer, who learnt cooking under his uncle at the celebrated Sree Padmanabhaswamy temple of Thiruvananthapuram, famous for its array of payasam, especially the pala payasam, used to make it with unhusked rice, the fresh milk of a cow that had just given birth and, of course, no sugar.

The Logic of Ancient Foods

In an opinion piece in *The New York Times*, Dr Haider Warraich, cardiologist with the Harvard Medical School and author of *State of the Heart: Exploring the History, Science and Future of Cardiac Disease* (St Martin's Press, 2019), puts up a singular question: 'Human evolution inadvertently led us into its labyrinthine lair. If that is true, is it possible for us to find our way out?' Can we have a chance at reversing these evolutionary mechanisms? The solution, he believes, is to transform our lifestyles, so that we can come up to speed with evolutionary mechanisms set in motion millennia ago: 'If we respect our evolution, adapt accordingly and follow evidence-based medical advice, we can revert it to a speck in the history of mankind.'[13]

That is the thought behind the rising interest in prehistoric eating habits. Anthropologists, archaeologists, doctors, nutritionists, celebrity chefs and movie stars are ditching sugar-rich modern diets to explore the human body's ancient connection to food. There has been an upsurge of interest in renewing seemingly forgotten traditional cooking skills and knowledge of foods. Wild food foraging and gathering edible plants, weeds and wildflowers—just as our hunter-gatherer ancestors did—is becoming a popular pastime in cities around the world. A growing number of groups are promoting the art and craft of foraging, with maps of fruit trees in the area, guided walks and workshops.

Restaurants around the world are offering foraged wild herbs, fruits and roots enriched with eco-friendly, integral flavours. They promote sustainable practices, indigenous produce and often work with professional foragers. Chef Prateek Sadhu, for instance, has worked in Michelin-starred restaurants across the world before coming back to India. He spent months travelling and exploring regional cuisines before opening his innovative fine-dining restaurant, Masque, in Mumbai, to showcase the plant-forward eating pattern that has been India's own since antiquity. And he forages ingredients himself, to prepare novel items.

Almost every other day, a new wonder diet becomes the latest fad. One such is the Palaeolithic or paleo diet, also known as the Stone Age diet, the hunter-gatherer diet or the caveman diet. This diet mimics how our prehistoric humans may have eaten, especially whole foods that people theoretically hunted or gathered. Advocates of the paleo diet reject any food that wasn't around at least 10,000 years ago, when agriculture began. Interest in plant-based diets is growing by the day. The low-fat diet, for instance, focuses on plenty of plant foods such as whole grains, fruits and vegetables, to help control the intake of fat, cholesterol, carbs and calories. The raw food diet is all about uncooked foods: anything that cannot be eaten raw is shunned.

If starvation has been a way of life in our distant past, why not a diet that follows the same biochemical processes in the body? Popularized by bestselling books and promoted by celebrities, the ketogenic or keto diet focuses on depleting the body of glucose, forcing it to burn fat and produce an alternate source of fuel called ketones. A typical keto diet cuts carbs (grains like rice and wheat, sugar and most fruits) down to less than

10 per cent of our daily intake. The rest is made up of fat (75 per cent) and protein (20 per cent). The keto diet leads to weight loss, but it has no shortage of detractors. Many find it worrisome that the diet restricts nutrient-rich foods supported by decades of research: high-fibre, unrefined carbohydrates, fruits and legumes, which are some of the most health-promoting foods on the planet and are not responsible for the epidemic of diabetes or obesity.

Forgotten Foods of the Past

Deep inside the spectacular biodiversity zone between the Maikal and Vindhya ranges of Chhattisgarh and Madhya Pradesh live the forest-dwelling Baigas, a tribe whose history goes back at least 20,000 years. The Baigas claim to be harbingers of the human race, the chosen people who were handcrafted by Bhagwan as the servants of the earth and the kings of the forests. Over the centuries, their language has faded away into oblivion (they speak a dialect of Hindi now), they seldom interact with others, avoid formal settlements, formal education, formal trade or work, and produce few implements. Art to them is basketry, decorative door carvings, tattoos, masks, and a rich world of songs, myths, lores and dances.

Recent studies link the Baigas to the Australian aborigines, by DNA and by their spoken language.[14] Officially, they are one of India's particularly vulnerable tribal groups, wracked by poverty and hunger, dissociated from all development processes, and displaced from their habitats by depleted forests and encroaching wildlife sanctuaries. Those who know them, respect them for their intimate knowledge of nature, complementary relationship with ecology and their time-tested nutrition. Dr Manjeet Kaur Bal has worked for long with tribes like the Baigas. As the leader of the Samerth Charitable Trust in Chhattisgarh, she has been helping them with their rights over the forest and land, basic entitlements, safe drinking water, hygiene, sanitation and nutrition.

Dr Bal knows why the Baigas never plough the earth or produce food from the same patch again and again. To the Baigas, the earth is their mother (Dharti Devi), ploughing would mean hurting the mother, and reaping food from the same patch of land again and again would make her weak. They, therefore, practise a type of cultivation called Bewar, by clearing the forests and being constantly on the move. As people of the forest, they take diverse and nutritious foods sourced from the forest. They eat coarse grains, especially minor millets like *kodo* and *kutki* that are now being recognized for their high-protein, high-fibre, mineral and antioxidant content.

Along with the world, India is experimenting with the nutritious small-seeded grasses called millets. Their origin goes back more than 10,000 years, when our ancestors started experimenting with curated grains. Hardy, climate-resilient, drought-tolerant and genetically rich, millets have grown with minimal human intervention. The seeds have been passed down from generations, especially as tribal staples in low-fertile, mountainous and rain-fed areas. Rich in vitamins, protein and fibre, millets are the new super cereals of our time. Prime Minister

Narendra Modi has been repeatedly saying: 'Barley, *jowar, ragi, kodo, sama,* millet, *sawa,* many such cereals were once part of our food. But gradually they disappeared from our plates. And this food was tagged with poverty.'[15]

Barley (*java*) is one of the earliest domesticated cereals of the world. It is what our ancient ancestors of Mohenjo-Daro, Harappa and Chanhudaro thrived on. It was also the first food of the Aryans (between 800–350 BCE). They parched and puffed barley grains (processes that break down carbs and proteins, making them easier to digest). They also ate fried barley cakes dipped in ghee and sweet barley flour cakes, and mixed powdered grains with water, ghee, milk, curd or even soma juice. Until 400 BCE, barley seems to have been the grain for all seasons—profane as well as sacred—gradually losing out to rice as the staple food of the Aryans. Barley is now largely used to make malt beer, but we can see a new ray of hope emerging with the identification of the health benefits of the ancient grain.

Scientists have found a high content of soluble fibres in barley, as compared with other cereal grains, that improve cholesterol levels in the blood, reduce bad LDL cholesterol and triglycerides, and keep the good HDL cholesterol levels up. Barley also has a lower GI compared with cereals like rice. Studies have shown that the consumption of barley improves insulin response, thus preventing quick and dangerous spikes in blood sugar. The myriad health benefits of barley have led to a surge of renewed interest in the ancient grain. Barley is now being regarded as a storehouse of phytochemicals, the naturally occurring antioxidants that are one of the most promising materials in animal diets.[16] One can only hope that the grain grabs public imagination once again and becomes a part of the modern Indian platter.

Coming back from the past is a bouquet of heirloom aromatic and coloured (owing to the deposition of a type of antioxidant in the bran layer) rice grains. These grains have remarkable nutritional potential (high-resistant starch, amylose, polyphenols and antioxidant content, as well as low GI), superior cooking qualities and blissful aroma. India has had more than 1,10,000 varieties of rice until the 1970s, lost largely in the wake of the Green Revolution, with its emphasis on yield rather than quality. Also, with the promotion of hybrid crops, many more are on the verge of extinction.

Since 2003, however, when the Government of India's Geographical Indications registry was set up, endangered varieties of fragrant rice are getting a new lease of life, with nearly 16–17 already on the list. For instance: Navara of Kerala, Kala Namak of Uttar Pradesh, Ambemohar of Maharashtra, Joha Saul of Assam, Gobindobhog of West Bengal and Chak-hao of Manipur are gaining considerable attention in the international market for their use in multinational cuisine as well as for their nutrition value. Many of these grains possess aroma and cooking qualities superior to the Basmati, elongate on cooking more than the Basmati and are more affordable than the Basmati.[17]

The earliest records of coloured rice—red, purple, black, brown, yellow and green—are found in the Taittiriya Samhita of the Yajur Veda (1500–800 BCE) as ritual offerings: black rice to Agni; red grains to

Brihaspati and Indra; yellow rice to Vishnu and so on. Archaeological evidence indicates aromatic rice (collectively called Basmati) evolved in northern India at least 8,000 years ago. While coloured grains were preferred by the founding fathers of ancient Ayurveda—Susruta, Charaka and Vagbhata, between 400 BCE and 700 CE—for their medicinal value, aromatic grains were chosen by the elite for their exclusive taste.[18]

In the last two decades, a flurry of studies have called for lifestyle changes and diet modification—less refined carbs and added sugars, more fibre-rich foods—to deal with the spiralling epidemics of obesity, diabetes and heart disease that stare us right in the face. Ancient whole grains have come to be regarded as doubly beneficial for us: gram for gram, these whole grains offer fewer carbs, better carbs, more protein and more beneficial fibres and micronutrients. It is high time these grains made their way back to the Indian platter, replacing the refined white rice.

The Devi Mahatmya

In the heart of Varanasi, the *Saptarishi Aarti* is on. Seven purohits chant in unison, some hold flaming lamps, some fan the ceremonial *chamara*, some clang cymbals, some ring the prayer bell, some beat the enormous *jaydhaak*—in tandem with your heartbeats. Wreaths of incense float up, the heady fragrance of flowers hang in the air, the crowd presses in. No one can enter the sanctum sanctorum, except the priests. And no one can block one of the four doorways leading to it. Through that door,

Kashi Vishwanath looks at his lady, Devi Annapurna, in her temple—at all times. Block that door at your own peril.

She is the queen-goddess of Kashi. At her temple, her golden idol rests against red Banarasi panels amidst intricately carved silver walls. An enormous three-decked bejewelled crown rests upon her head, layers and layers of jewellery cover her torso. In one hand, she holds a golden ladle of rice like a sceptre, and in the other, a pot. Her three eyes look straight at you, benign and smiling. When you visit her temple, if she wills, you get a fistful of sacred rice wrapped in crimson cloth. Her prasad, on the special day around Diwali, are coins.

With Devi Annapurna, the instant association is with her namesake, *anna* or rice: in her temple, there is free distribution of rice every day. As the legend goes, her husband once negated the importance of food, citing it as a cosmic illusion, or *maya*. The Devi decided to teach him a lesson: she made herself invisible. With her, all food and nourishment vanished from the earth, a great famine visited and people started to die of hunger. Realizing his grave mistake, her husband begged for rice as alms from her. The Devi relented.

She is an aspect of Devi Adishakti, the universal primal force: a goddess of food, nourishment and prosperity. You would expect her to be served a majestic fare as naivedya, but she partakes modest meals. Saag, the humblest of leafy vegetables, with plenty of vitamins and minerals but nothing to write home about, is one of her favourite foods. At her temple, as part of the free lunch prasad for all devotees, you get a simple platter of rice, dal (sometimes the South Indian *sambaar* dal), sabzi, pickles, curd, papad and sweets. Rice with roasted black sesame seeds is served quite often.

What is the message of nutrition concealed in Devi Annapurna's prasad? It is to consume foods that strengthen your immune system, fight inflammation, keep your system cool and protect you from diseases—from common cold and diabetes, to heart disease and cancers. Take spinach, for instance: research shows that most of the carbs in spinach consist of healthy dietary fibre and contain a unique blend of bioactive components including resistant starches (which protect against a range of diseases, including colon cancer, diabetes and obesity), vitamins, minerals, phytochemicals (safeguard cells against damage and help regulate hormones) and antioxidants (prevent or slow cell damage).

Modern science is catching up with the wisdom of Devi Annapurna. Research shows that spinach contains antioxidants that suppress inflammation in our immune cells. And some of these can also be stored in the body, building up a reserve. Beta-carotene (red-orange pigment) in spinach converts into vitamin A (retinol) in the body which helps improve our vision, promotes healthy skin and develops a strong immune system. Antioxidants like lutein, which increases in cooked spinach, improves age-related vision problem—the leading cause of blindness in India. Lutein has been found to be significantly low in the bloodstream of people with heart disease. Some research suggests that low blood levels of lutein and carotenoids are linked to blood sugar problems.

In July 2021, scientists from the Stanford School of

Medicine announced the results of their study conducted on the impact of different diets on the microbiome and health.[19] Topping the list are fermented foods—from yogurt to pickles—which can increase microbiome diversity and lower inflammation. The credit goes to vitamin K, a crucial component for wound healing and healthy bones. Spinach, fermented food like curd, pickles, sambaar and sesame rice—served at the Annapurna temple—get the thumbs up for being high on vitamin K, as well as for being gut-friendly and anti-inflammatory. Follow a similar diet and you might just reduce your risk of developing diabetes, arthritis, heart disease, osteoarthritis and a range of other disorders.

Very different from Devi Annapurna is Devi Durga, the goddess of life, power and strength, with 10 mighty hands, many names, many persona and many facets. Born of a ball of fire from the combined energy of the gods to kill a fearsome demon, she herself is the colour of flame. Riding a lion, as she enters the battlefield of good versus evil, her crown kisses the sky, her hands wield weapons of destruction and her three eyes emit fire. The earth trembles with every footstep and the universe cowers at her battle cry: she is Adya Mahashakti, the first among the conscious forces of the cosmos that dominate all existence.

Yet, during her autumnal sojourn to earth every year, she is offered the most rustic of fares: *panta bhaat* or leftover rice soaked overnight—technically, submerged in an inch of water and covered with a light piece of fabric. This lightly fermented grub is then consumed the next morning, or as fillers between meals, typically with green or roasted chilly, salt and spinach (saag), sometimes with lime, a few slices of onion, a bit of mustard oil, pickles, curry or fried fish. In the competitive world of TV cooking, it is now being called 'Smoked Rice Water'.[20] The Bengali proverb, however, that goes with this extremely humble dish is: *'Noon ante panta phuraay'*, meaning extremely straitened circumstances.

Called panta bhaat in Bengal (and Bangladesh), *poita bhat* in Assam, *pakhala bhaat* in Odisha, *bore bhat* in Chhattisgarh, *paani bhaat* in Jharkhand, and *pazhaya sadam* and *pazham kanji* in southern India, it is a centuries-old recipe, the commonest dish prepared from leftover food alone. Panta is not just a mark of subaltern gastronomy of rural India, it is the food of the original inhabitants of South Asia—the Proto-Australoid aborigines—who cooked once a day, most likely in the evenings. Just as the tribes of Central India, the Baigas too drink rice water which they call *torani*, with added flavours. The question is: why does a prodigiously powerful Aryan goddess choose the food of the poor, that too the food of the people who were vanquished and displaced by the Aryans?

The answers are based in science: panta bhaat has more essential micronutrients than fresh rice, reports a study by agricultural biotechnologists of Assam Agricultural University, Jorhat.[21] The anti-nutritional components of rice (like phytic acid) make it difficult for many of the nutrients present in the grain to be absorbed by the human body. This changes in panta bhaat with the passage of fermentation time. Nutrients like magnesium, calcium, iron and zinc increase while phytic acid goes down. Even more exciting research is being reported from AIIMS, Bhubaneswar.[22] Panta bhaat contains beneficial short-chain fatty acids that boost immunity and regulate inflammation.

Let's come to the fiercest goddess of them all: Kali. Naked, dark as the night, bedecked with freshly cut human arms and heads, and tongue lolling with blood, she roams cremation grounds. In her battle with demons, she roars, laughs boisterously and dances with such abandon that the demons faint. That raucous abandon is mirrored among her devotees at the Kalighat temple in Kolkata. Every day, as the serpentine queue reaches the doorway to her sanctum sanctorum, people who looked perfectly normal just a few minutes ago suddenly start shouting 'Jai Ma'. Some bang their head on the walls of her chamber, some burst into wild gesticulation, some fall to the ground in a swoon. The enormously tall goddess looks on with her three eyes—unsmiling.

What food does Kali prefer? The answer should be obvious, for animal sacrifices still continue at the temple. But she, too, has a penchant for common people's food: the ubiquitous greenish-purple stem of *kochu shaak* (taro or *arbi saag*). Essentially a village food, cooked and consumed largely by women, taro is rich in micronutrients like magnesium, potassium, phosphorus, and vitamins C, B and E. It especially offers protection against anaemia—the bane of Indian women. Molecular biologists are now exploring valuable bioactive molecules in taro corms, which are effective against cancer, cell damage, inflammation and metabolic dysfunctions like diabetes. They are calling for the popularization of taro intake as a dietary intervention strategy to improve overall health and as a supportive therapy for cancer.

What's common in the foods of the three prime goddesses of the Hindu pantheon is that they all advocate cooling foods that fight inflammation and boost immunity. These are also great eating patterns, because chronic low-grade inflammation is linked to a range of disorders: diabetes, heart disease, arthritis, dementia to cancer. In the last decade, a number of experimental studies have shown that components of foods or beverages impact the inflammatory processes. While refined carbs, fried foods, sugar-sweetened beverages, red and processed meat are pro-inflammatory, coloured and green leafy vegetables, nuts and seeds, fatty fish, fruits, green tea and turmeric are anti-inflammatory. It's a coming together of religion, ancient wisdom and modern science. And the nutritional message is the same: cool the flames burning inside you.

The Last Message

The offering of food by Sujata was a turning point in the Buddha's journey. It was the food that restored his health. My history textbook never told me that the Buddha died of food, too. He was at the city of Pave, Padrauna in present-day Uttar Pradesh, when Cunda, a blacksmith of the town, invited him for a meal of rice, cakes and *sukaramaddava* or boar's delight. Scholars are not sure if it was a boar's tender flesh or some kind of edible mushroom. Whatever it might have been, the Buddha realized that there was something wrong with it. After eating some of it, he ordered the rest to be buried in a pit. Shortly afterwards, he became violently ill. He still walked six miles to Kushinagar, gave his last admonitions to thousands of followers and was laid to his last rest.

Is there a message in his death? I would think so, even if a symbolic one: that the line between life and death is mercilessly thin and that the man who took such meticulous care of food and health—his own and his monks—should be gone by one wrong food. And the story tells me to wake up and be vigilant. Today's sukaramaddava can very well be the silent killer of this book: sugar.

Acknowledgements

No book is complete without acknowledging those who make it possible. My first debt of gratitude goes to Aroon Purie, editor-in-chief of the India Today Group. This book began life as a cover story for *India Today* magazine in November 2018 under his guidance.

I still remember the storm of discussions in our newsroom, with reporters recounting well-hidden manifestations of diabetes among the political class in India. The editor had pointed out that there were about 33 million people with diabetes in India the last time *India Today* did a cover story on diabetes in 2003. This figure had climbed to 82 million by 2018. What was going on? It felt like an apocalyptic scene, driven by sugar. It was a story that had to be told.

This was the time when a study led by AIIMS, Delhi, revealed that diabetes had shot up in India by about 200 per cent between 1990 and 2016. Around this time, the Ayushman Bharat Pradhan Mantri Jan Arogya Yojana was being rolled out across India. I still remember Dr Vinod Paul, member of NITI Aayog and architect of the scheme, telling me how the first beneficiary turned out to be a young woman in a Chhattisgarh village, who had no clue that she had uncontrolled diabetes. 'Nearly 70 per cent people with diabetes in India don't,' he had explained.

My special appreciation goes to my friend and former art director of *India Today* magazine, Madhu Bhaskar, who designed the delightful cover of this book. It gives me great pleasure to thank Dr Devi Shetty, for writing the Foreword. Without the conversations I have had with him on the idea of eating against nature, this book would not have been possible. I would also like to take this opportunity to thank Dr Ambrish Mithal, Dr Nikhil Tandon, Dr Naresh Trehan, Dr Arvind Kumar, Dr Anoop Misra, Dr Rajesh Malhotra, Dr V. Mohan, Dr K.S. Reddy and Dr Vinod Paul, whose friendship, time and patient teaching have helped me navigate the gap between expert knowledge and popular understandings of the body and disease always. A large thank you to Rupa Publications for the keen interest the house takes in health non-fiction, especially to Yamini Chowdhury, senior commissioning editor, for her upbeat support always.

Finally, I would like to thank my family, to whom I owe a great deal. To my late father H.C. Datta, who believed in me more than I did. An enormous thanks to my sister, Gargi, for always listening to me patiently and for being with me every step of the way. And finally to my mother, Gayatri, for her endless love and support.

Notes

Chapter 1: An Inheritance of Sugar

1. For a commentary on Bengali eccentricity, see Datta-Ray, Sunanda K. and Indrajit Hazra, *Calcutta Then: Kolkata Now*, Roli Books, Delhi, 2018.
2. Das Gupta, Minakshie et al., *The Calcutta Cookbook: A Treasury of Over 200 Recipes from Pavement to Palace*, Penguin, New Delhi, 1995, p. 352.
3. Sen, Colleen Taylor, 'Sandesh: An Emblem of Bengaliness', in *Milk: Beyond the Dairy*, H. Walker (ed.), Proceedings of the Oxford Symposium on Food and Cookery, Prospect Books, Devon, 1999, pp. 300–08.
4. Lévi-Strauss, Claude, *Totémism*, Rodney Needham (trans.), *Totemism*, Beacon Press, Boston, 1963, p. 89.
5. Kapoor, Hansika and James C. Kaufman, 'Meaning-Making through Creativity during COVID-19', *Frontiers in Psychology*, 18 December 2020, pp. 1–8, https://doi.org/10.3389/fpsyg.2020.595990.
6. Creswell, Julie, 'I Just Need the Comfort: Processed Foods Make a Pandemic Comeback', *The New York Times*, 7 April 2020, https://nyti.ms/3hYDlCQ. Accessed on 20 October 2021.
7. Spence, Charles, 'Comfort food: A review', *International Journal of Gastronomy and Food Science*, 9 (2017): 105–09.
8. Locher, J. et al., 'Comfort foods: An exploratory journey into the social and emotional significance of food', *Food and Foodways*, 13(4), October–December 2005, (273–97), p. 750.
9. Haldar, J., *Bengal Sweets*, Industry Publishers Ltd, Calcutta, Fifth edition, 1948, p. 2.

10. Rufus, Anneli, 'How comfort foods work like Prozac: The psychology behind why we turn to fatty staples like French fries and fried chicken when life gets rough', *Salon*, 23 June 2011, https://bit.ly/3tNDazJ. Accessed on 20 October 2021.
11. Kandiah, J. et al., 'Stress influences appetite and comfort food preferences in college women', *Nutrition Research*, 26(3), March 2006, pp. 118–23.
12. Gulati, Seema and Anoop Misra, 'Sugar Intake, Obesity, and Diabetes in India', *Nutrients*, 6(12) (December 2014): 5955–74.
13. Mohan, Viswanathan et al., 'Are excess carbohydrates the main link to diabetes & its complications in Asians?' *Indian J Med Res.*, November 2018, 148(5): 531–38, doi: 10.4103/ijmr.IJMR_1698_18.
14. Sharma, M. et al., 'A comparison of the Indian diet with the EAT-Lancet reference diet', *BMC Public Health*, Vol. 20 (2020), p. 812.
15. Willett, W. et al., 'Food in the Anthropocene: the EAT–Lancet Commission on healthy diets from sustainable food systems', *The Lancet*, 2019, 6736: 3–49. 393: 447–92.
16. Mintz, Sidney W., *Sweetness and Power: The Place of Sugar in Modern History*, Viking Penguin, New York, 1985.
17. Abbott, Elizabeth, *Sugar: A Bittersweet History*, Duckworth Overlook, New York and London, 2009; Walvin, James, *Sugar: The World Corrupted: From Slavery to Obesity*, Hatchette, London, 2017; Taubes, Gary, *The Case Against Sugar*, Alfred A. Knopf, New York, 2016.
18. Kearns, C.E. et al., 'Sugar Industry and Coronary Heart Disease Research: A Historical Analysis of Internal Industry Documents', *Journal of American Medical Association, JAMA Intern Med.*, 176(11): 1680–85, doi:10.1001/jamainternmed.2016.5394.
19. Tapsell, L.C. et al., 'Foods, nutrients, and dietary patterns: Interconnections and implications for dietary guidelines', *Adv Nutr*, 7(30), 2016: 445–54.
20. Tagore, Rabindranath, *Jibansmriti*, Visva Bharati Press, Calcutta, 1959.
21. *Nolen gur* means new jaggery in Bengal. It is extracted from date palm trees during winter.
22. *Mangal Kavya*, a vast body of narrative verses dedicated to popular gods and goddesses and composed by authors from various regions of Bengal (13–18 CE), also sang paeans to the

food cooked by the women of the times.
23 *Sandesh* is a Bangla children's magazine, first published by Upendrakishore Roychowdhury (1863–1915 CE) in 1913. He was a writer, musicologist, artist, publisher, editor and printer of repute. After him, *Sandesh* was edited by his son, Sukumar Ray, grandson Satyajit Ray and great grandson, Sandip Ray.
24 Doctor, Vikram and Writanker Mukherjee, 'The great rosogolla revolt: When a Bengal CM banned Bengali sweets', *The Economic Times*, 25 July 2015, https://bit.ly/3ML7X8L. Accessed on 20 October 2021.
25 Eaton, R.M., *The Rise of Islam and the Bengal Frontier, 1204–1760*, University of California Press, Berkeley, 1993.
26 Chattopadhyaya, Annapurna, *The People and Culture of Bengal: A Study in Origins*, Vol. I (part-2), Firma KLM Private Ltd, Kolkata, 2002.
27 For instance, Bhatta Bhavadeva, an eleventh century CE scholar and royal official of Bengal, wrote in his text on expiatory rites, *Prayaschitta Prakaranam*, that the prohibitions of eating fish and meat for Brahmins existed only on certain festive days.
28 Ray, Niharranjan, *History of the Bengali People: From Earliest Times to the Fall of the Sena Dynasty*, John W. Wood (trans.), Orient Longman, Calcutta, 1994.
29 The Nastika schools do not accept the authority of the Vedas: the system of the four castes and the superiority of the Brahmins.
30 O'Malley, L.S.S. and Monmohan Chakravarti, *Bengal District Gazetteer*, The Bengal Secretariat Book Depot, Calcutta, 1912, pp. 25–42.
31 Achaya, K.T., *A Historical Dictionary of Indian Food*, Oxford University Press, Delhi, 2001, p. 128.
32 The secretive and esoteric philosophy of Tantra, which began to spread all over India around fifth–sixth century CE, emphasized five Ms, also known as *panchamakara* or *panchatattva*: *madya* (amrita), *mamsa* (meat), *matsya* (fish), *mudra* (gesture) and *maithuna* (sexual intercourse).
33 Achaya, K.T., *Indian Food: A Historical Companion*, Oxford University Press, Delhi, 1994, p. 125.
34 Banerji, Chitrita, *Life and Food in Bengal*, Penguin Books, New Delhi, 2005, p. 23.

35 Ray, Utsa, *Culinary Culture in Colonial India: A Cosmopolitan Platter and the Middle-Class*, Cambridge University Press, Delhi, 2015, p. 151.
36 Chakravarty, Taponath, *Food and Drink in Ancient Bengal*, Firma KL Mukhpadhyay, Calcutta, 1959, pp. 7–19.
37 Sandhyakar Nandi (c. 1084–1155 CE), a poet of Pala Dynasty, in his Sanskrit *kavya* (epic), *Ramacharitam*.
38 Sen, Colleen Taylor, 'Sandesh: An emblem of Bengaliness', in *Milk: Beyond the dairy*, H. Walker (ed.), Prospect Books, Devon, 2000, p. 300.
39 Ghosh, Suchandra and Sayantani Pal, 'Everyday Life in Early Bengal', in *History of Bangladesh, Early Bengal in Regional Perspectives up to c.1200 CE*, Vol. II, Abdul Momin Chowdhury and Ranabir Chakravarti (eds), Asiatic Society of Bangladesh, Dhaka, 2018, p. 21.
40 Grose, F., *A Voyage to the East Indies*, Vol. II, S. Hooper, London, 1772, p. 234.
41 Sengupta, Nirmal, *Traditional Knowledge in Modern India: Preservation, Promotion, Ethical Access and Benefit Sharing Mechanisms*, Springer, Delhi, 2019, p. 111.
42 Unknown, *Pakrajeshwar*, N.L. Sil, Kolkata, 1831.
43 Mukhopadhay, Bipradas, *Pak-Pratali*, Metcalfe Press, Calcutta, 1898.
44 Dasgupta, S. et al., *Heritage Tourism: An Anthropological Journey to Bishnupur*, Mittal Publications, Delhi, 2009.
45 Banerjee, Milinda, 'Gods in a Democracy: State of Nature, Postcolonial Politics, and Bengali Mangalkabyas', in *The Postcolonial World*, G. Jyotsna Singh and David D. Kim (eds), Routledge, New York, 2017, p. 195.
46 Krondl, Michael, *Sweet Invention: A History of Dessert*, Chicago Review Press, Chicago, 2011.
47 Mukhopadhyay, Ashoke Kumar, 'Sweets of Kolkata', 1999, http//lokfolk.blogspot.in/2009/05/sweetsofkolkata. Accessed on 11 April 2022.
48 Goldstein, D., *The Oxford Companion to Sugar and Sweets*, Oxford University Press, 2015.
49 Nandy, S.C., *The History of the Cossimbazar Raj in the Nineteenth Century*, Vol. I, P.K. Roy, Calcutta, 1957.

50 Sengupta, Rimli, 'The Legends Behind Bengal's Famous Sweets', *Outlook Traveller*, 15 October 2021, https://bit.ly/3xR7j4w. Accessed on 24 April 2022.
51 Karkaria, Bachi, *Flurys of Calcutta: The Cake That Walked*, Flurys, Calcutta, 2007, pp. 1–10.
52 Charles, R., 'Diabetes in the tropics', *British Medical Journal*, 1907; 19: 1051–64.
53 Swami Vivekananda, *The East and the West*, Advaita Ashram, Mayavati, Uttarakhand, 2002.
54 Tandon, Nikhil et al., 'The increasing burden of diabetes and variations among the states of India: the Global Burden of Disease Study 1990–2016', *The Lancet*, December 2018, 6 (12): E1352–62.
55 Misra, P. et al., 'A review of the epidemiology of diabetes in rural India', *Diabetes Research and Clinical Practice*, April 2011 (92): 303–11.
56 Ravikanth, Lavanya and K.S. Kavi Kumar, 'Caught in the Net: Fish Consumption Patterns of Coastal Regions in India', Working paper 110/2015, Madras School of Economics, Chennai, June 2015, pp. 3–8.

Chapter 2: Should You Be Afraid of Sugar?

1 Yudkin, John, *Pure, White and Deadly: How Sugar Is Killing Us and What We Can Do to Stop It*, Penguin, London, 1972, 1986, p. viii.
2 *Nature*, 156, 471 (1945), https://doi.org/10.1038/156471c0.
3 Nernpermpisooth, N. et al., 'Obesity Alters the Peripheral Circadian Clock in the Aorta and Microcirculation. Microcirculation', *National Library of Science*, 2015, 22(4): 257–66.
4 Leslie, Ian, 'The sugar conspiracy', *The Guardian*, 7 April 2016, https://bit.ly/37bDP6R. Accessed on 14 April 2022.
5 'Sugar: The Bitter Truth', a lecture by Dr Robert H. Lustig (Professor Emeritus, the Department of Pediatrics and the Center for Obesity Assessment, Study and Treatment at the University of California, San Francisco, California) on 26 May 2009; presented by UCSF's Osher Center for Integrative Medicine as part of the Mini Medical School for the public lecture series on 'Current Controversies in Nutrition: Letting Science Be the Guide'. The University of California Television uploaded the video on YouTube

on 31 July 2009. To see the video, visit: https://www.youtube.com/watch?v=dBnniua6-oM. Accessed on 11 April 2022.

6. Professor Walter C. Willett is a physician and nutrition researcher. Currently, he is the Fredrick John Stare Professor of Epidemiology and Nutrition at the Harvard School of Public Health. He was the chair (1991–2017) of the Department of Nutrition at Harvard. Dr Frank B. Hu is the chair of the Department of Nutrition and the Fredrick John Stare Professor of Nutrition and Epidemiology at Harvard T.H. Chan School of Public Health, and professor of Medicine at the Harvard Medical School. Dr David S. Ludwig is a professor in the Department of Nutrition at Harvard T.H. Chan School of Public Health, and director of the New Balance Foundation Obesity Prevention Center at Boston Children's Hospital. Dr Kelly D. Bromwell is the co-founder and former director of Yale University's Rudd Center for Food Policy & Obesity.

7. Kearns, C. et al., 'Sugar Industry and Coronary Heart Disease Research: A Historical Analysis of Internal Industry Documents', *JAMA Intern Med*, November 2016, 176(11):1680–85.

8. Datta, Damayanti, 'Why eggs are good for you: New study shows eggs aren't the devils that increase risk of heart disease', *India Today*, 10 November 2017, https://bit.ly/3Kw1lK4. Accessed on 11 April 2022.

9. World Health Organization, 'Diet, nutrition and the prevention of chronic diseases: Report of a Joint WHO/FAO Expert Consultation', WHO, Geneva, 2003.

10. 'Global study finds diet high in poor-quality carbohydrates increases heart disease and death', U of T News, https://bit.ly/3roZVt6. Accessed on 14 April 2022.

11. Jenkins, David J.A. et al., 'Glycemic Index, Glycemic Load, and Cardiovascular Disease and Mortality', *N Engl J Med*, 384 (April 2021):1312–22.

12. Lustig, Robert H., *Sugar Has 56 Names: A Shopper's Guide*, Hudson Street Press, New York, 2013.

13. 'Learn to recognize the 56 different names for sugar', RobertLustig.com, https://robertlustig.com/56-names-of-sugar/.

14. Yudkin, John, *Pure, White and Deadly: How Sugar Is Killing Us and What We Can Do to Stop It*, Penguin, London, 1972, 1986, p. 149.

Chapter 3: Blooms, Bees and Sugar, Please

1. Neumayer, Erwin, *Lines on Stone: The Prehistoric Rock Art of India*, Manohar Publishers, New Delhi, 1993.
2. Pager, H., 'Rock Paintings in Southern Africa Showing Bees and Honey Hunting', *Bee Worlds*, June 1973, 54 (2), doi.org/10.1080/0005772X.1973.11097456.
3. Whitley, David S. (ed), *Handbook of Rock Art Research*, Rowman & Littlefield, Boston, 2001.
4. Dr Devi Prasad Shetty, MS, FRCS, is a cardiac surgeon and entrepreneur. He is the chairman and founder of Narayana Health, one of India's largest hospital chains, headquartered in Bengaluru, India.
5. 'Global Nutrition Report: Shining a light to spur action on nutrition', Development Initiatives Bristol, UK, 2018.
6. Shetty, Dr Devi Prasad, 'The worst offence against the body is eating against nature', *India Today*, 25 May 2012, https://bit.ly/3JXknYR. Accessed on 15 April 2022.
7. Goulson, Dave, *A Sting in the Tale: My Adventures with Bumblebees*, Jonathan Cape, London, 2013.
8. Wallberg, Andreas et al., 'A worldwide survey of genome sequence variation provides insight into the evolutionary history of the honeybee Apis mellifera', *Nature Genetics*, October 2014, 46(10):1081–88, doi: 10.1038/ng.3077.
9. Wheeler, A.L. et al., 'The Expensive-Tissue Hypothesis: The Brain and the Digestive System in Human and Primate Evolution', *Current Anthropology*, April 1995, 36 (2): 199–221.
10. Baschetti, R., 'Evolutionary Physiology Shows the Need for an Unprecedented Study on Sugar', *Clin Nutr ESPEN*, June 2019, 31:23–27, doi: 10.1016/j.clnesp.2019.03.012.
11. Pollan, Michael, *The Omnivore's Dilemma: A Natural History of Four Meals*, Penguin Press, New York, 2006.
12. Larbey, Cynthia et al., 'Cooked Starchy Food in Hearths ca. 120 kya and 65 kya (MIS 5e and MIS 4) from Klasies River Cave, South Africa', *Journal of Human Evolution*, June 2019, 131(20): 210–27, DOI:10.1016/j.jhevol.2019.03.015.
13. Arranz-Otaegui, Amaia et al, 'Archaeobotanical Evidence Reveals the Origins of Bread 14,400 Years Ago in Northeastern Jordan',

Proceedings of the National Academy of Sciences of the USA, July 2018, 115(31):7925–30, doi: 10.1073/pnas.1801071115.

14. Wrangham, Richard, *Catching Fire: How Cooking Made Us Human,* Profile Books, London, 2009.
15. Crittenden, A.N., 'The Importance of Honey Consumption in Humans Evolution', *Food and Foodways,* October 2011, 19 (4): 257–73, doi:10.1080/07409710.2011.630618.
16. Roffet-Salque, Mélanie, 'Widespread Exploitation of the Honeybee by Early Neolithic Farmers', *Nature,* January 2015, 534 (7607), doi:10.1038/nature18451.
17. Ghurye, G.S., *Indian Acculturation: Agastya and Skanda,* Popular Prakashan, Mumbai, 1977.
18. Sato, T., *Sugar in the Social Life of Medieval Islam,* Brill, Leiden, 2015.
19. Jones, Horace Leonard, *The Geography of Strabo* (translated), Harvard University Press, Cambridge, 1932.
20. Nunn, J.F., *Ancient Egyptian Medicine,* University of Oklahoma Press, Oklahoma, 1996.
21. Rajasekharan, S. and G.S. Raju, 'Certain Concepts of "Prameha" (diabetes) in Ayurveda (Indian System of Medicine) with special Reference to the Relationship between Ancient Indian and Modern Thoughts, Ancient Science of Life', *Ancient Science of Life,* April 1982, II (1): 17–22, https://pubmed.ncbi.nlm.nih.gov/22556917/. Accessed on 12 March 2022.
22. Das, Sukta, 'Prevention of Diabetes–A Historical Note', *Indian Journal of History of Science,* August 2013.
23. Das, Sukta, 'Perception of Food and Nutrition and Dietary Recommendation in Health and Disease: Focus on Caraka-Susruta Samhitas', *Indian Journal of History of Science,* March 2015, 50 (1): 131–47, DOI: 10.16943/ijhs/2015/v50i1/48116.
24. Lunia, B.N., *Evolution of Indian Culture from the Earliest Times to the Present Day,* Lakshmi Narayan Agarwal, Agra, 1955, pp. 73–108.
25. Robyt, J.F., *Essentials of Carbohydrate Chemistry,* Springer: Verlag New York-Berlin-Heidelberg, 1998.
26. Munro, J.H.A., 'Oriental Spices and Their Costs in Medieval Cuisine: Luxuries or Necessities?' (University College, Toronto, lecture in 1988) in *Money, Markets and Trade in Late Medieval Europe: Essays in Honour of John H. A. Munro,* L. Armstrong et al. (eds), Leiden, Boston, 2007, p. 32.

27 Mintz, Sidney W., *Sweetness and Power: The Place of Sugar in Modern History*, Viking: New York, 1986.
28 Basu, Sanjay et al., 'Estimation of Global Insulin Use for Type 2 Diabetes, 2018–30: A Microsimulation Analysis', *The Lancet*, November 2018, 7(1): 25–33, doi.org/10.1016/S2213-8587(18): 30303-6.
29 Eaton, S.B. et al., 'Stone Agers in the Fast Lane: Chronic Degenerative Diseases in Evolutionary Perspective', *Am J Med*, April 1988, 84 (4): 739–49.

Chapter 4: Sweet Cravings of a Stone Age Brain

1 Richmond, B.G. et al., 'The Upper Limb of Paranthropus boisei from Ileret, Kenya', *Journal of Human Evolution*, February 2020, IF3.895, DOI: 10.1016/j.jhevol.2019.102727.
2 Quinn, R.L. et al., 'Contracting Eastern African C4 Grasslands during the Extinction of *Paranthropus boisei*', *Nature*, 2021, 11:7164, https://doi.org/10.1038/s41598-021-86642-z.
3 Cerling, T.E. et al., 'Diet of Paranthropus boisei in the early Pleistocene of East Africa', *Proceedings of the National Academy of Sciences*, 2011, doi: 10.1073/pnas.1104627108.
4 Leakey, L.S.B. et al., 'A New Species of the Genus *Homo* from Olduvai Gorge', *Nature*, 1964, 202: 7–9.
5 Ungar, P.S. et al., 'Dental Microwear and Diet of the Plio-Pleistocene Hominin Paranthropus boise', *PLoS ONE*, 2008, 3(4): e2044, doi:10.1371/journal.pone.0002044.
6 Hardy, Karen et al., 'The Importance of Dietary Carbohydrate in Human Evolution', *The Quarterly Review of Biology*, September 2015, 90 (3): 251–68, doi.org/10.1086/682587.
7 Shanahan, Mike, *Gods, Wasps and Stranglers: The Secret History and Redemptive Future of Fig Trees*, Chelsea Green Publishing, Chelsea, 2018, Chapter 2.
8 M.E. Kislev et al., 'Early domesticated fig in the Jordan Valley', *Science*, June 2006, 2: 312(5778):1372–74, doi: 10.1126/science.1125910.
9 Robertson, Tracey M. et al., 'Starchy Carbohydrates in a Healthy Diet: The Role of the Humble Potato', *Nutrients*, 14 November 2018, 10(11): 1764. doi:10.3390/nu10111764.

10 Wrangham, R. et al., 'Cooking as a Biological Trait', *Comp Biochem Physiol,* September 2003,136(1): 35–46, doi: 10.1016/s1095-6433(03)00020-5.

11 Baldwin, M.W. et al., 'Evolution of Sweet Taste Perception in Hummingbirds by Transformation of the Ancestral Umami Receptor', *Science,* August 2014, 345 (6199): 929–33, doi: 10.1126/science.1255097.

12 Schweiger, Kerstin et al., 'Sweet Taste Antagonist Lactisole Administered in Combination with Sucrose, But Not Glucose, Increases Energy Intake and Decreases Peripheral Serotonin in Male Subjects', *Nutrients,* 2020, 12 (10): 3133, doi: 10.3390/nu12103133.

13 Briški, F. et al., 'Environmental Microbiology', *Physical Sciences Reviews,* 2017, 2(11): 20160118, doi.org/10.1515/psr-2016-0118.

14 Hull, P., 'Life in the Aftermath of Mass Extinctions', *Curr Biol,* 2015; 25: R941–52.

15 Johnson, R.J. et al., 'Fructose Metabolism as a Common Evolutionary Pathway of Survival Associated with Climate Change, Food Shortage and Droughts', *The Association for the Publication of the Journal of Internal Medicine,* 2019, doi: 10.1111/joim.12993.

16 Berridge, K.C. et al., 'Dissecting Components of Reward: "liking," "wanting," and learning', *Current Opinion in Pharmacology,* January 2009, 9(1):65–73. DOI: 10.1016/j.coph.2008.12.014.

17 Berridge, Kent C. et al., 'The Tempted Brain Eats: Pleasure and desire circuits in obesity and eating disorders', *Brain Res,* 2 September 2010, 1350: 43–64, DOI:10.1016/j.brainres.2010.04.003.

18 Wiss, D.A. et al., 'Sugar Addiction: From Evolution to Revolution', *Front. Psychiatry,* 7 November 2018, 9:545, doi: 10.3389/fpsyt.2018.00545.

19 Bragulat, V. et al., 'Food-Related Odor Probes of Brain Reward Circuits during Hunger: A Pilot fMRI Study', *Obesity,* September 2012, 18 (8): 156–671, DOI: 10.1038/oby.2010.57.

20 Stewart, P.C. and Erica Gross, 'Plate Shape and Colour Interact to Influence Taste and Quality Judgments', *Flavour,* 2013, 2 (27), DOI: 10.1186/2044-7248-2-27.

21 Spence, Charles and Betina Piqueras-Fiszman, *The Perfect Meal: The Multisensory Science of Food and Dining,* Wiley-Blackwell, Oxford, 2014, pp. 12–22.

22 'How Does Eating Affect Your Blood Sugar?' *healthline*, https://bit.ly/3JImwr1. Accessed on 12 April 2022.
23 Wasserman, D.A., 'Four Grams of Glucose', *American Journal of Physiology-Endocrinology and Metabolism*, September 2012, 296 (1): E11–E21, doi: 10.1152/ajpendo.90563.2008.
24 Sugar cane Statistics, Report of ICAR-Sugar Institute Breeding Institute, India, June 2021.
25 Division of Public Health Services, New Hampshire Department of Health and Human Services, Health Promotion in Motion; United States Department of Agriculture (USDA) Sugar and Sweetener Outlook data.
26 Lowe, M.R. et al., 'Hedonic Hunger: a new dimension of appetite?' *Physiol Behav*, July 2007, 91(4):432–39, doi: 10.1016/j.physbeh.2007.04.006.
27 Darwin, Charles, *The Expression of the Emotions in Man and Animals*, John Murray, London, 1872.
28 Olds, J. and P. Milner, 'Positive Reinforcement Produced by Electrical Stimulation of Septal Area and Other Regions of Rat Brain', *J Comp Physiol Psychol*, December 1954, 47(6): 419–27.
29 Kringelbach, M.L., 'Emotion', in *The Oxford Companion to the Mind, 2nd edition*, R.L. Gregory (ed), Oxford University Press, Oxford, UK, 2004, pp. 287–90.
30 Lieberman, Daniel E., 'Evolution's Sweet Tooth', *The New York Times*, 5 June 2012, https://nyti.ms/3rcF1xm. Accessed on 27 October 2021; Lieberman, Daniel E., *The Story of the Human Body: Evolution, Health, and Disease*, Pantheon Books, New York, 2013.

Chapter 5: What Sugar Really Does to You

1 Tandon, Nikhil et al., 'The increasing burden of diabetes and variations among the states of India: The Global Burden of Disease Study 1990–2016', *The Lancet*, December 2018, 6 (12): E1352–E1362, https://doi.org/10.1016/S2214-109X(18)30387-5.
2 Ramachandran, A. et al., 'Increasing expenditure on health care incurred by diabetic subjects in a developing country: A study from India', Diabetes Care, February 2007, 30(2): 252–6, doi: 10.2337/dc06-0144.
3 Measured as Disability-Adjusted Life-Years (DALY), where one

year of healthy life lost is measured per 100,000 population (Tandon, Nikhil et al., 'The increasing burden of diabetes and variations among the states of India: The Global Burden of Disease Study 1990–2016', *The Lancet*, December 2018, 6 (12): E1352–E1362).
4. Zimmet, P.Z., 'Diabetes and its drivers: the largest epidemic in human history?' *Clin Diabetes Endocrinol*, 2017, 3 (1), https://doi.org/10.1186/s40842-016-0039-3.
5. Ibid.
6. Saeedi, P. et al., IDF Diabetes Atlas Committee, 'Global and regional diabetes prevalence estimates for 2019 and projections for 2030 and 2045: Results from the International Diabetes Federation Diabetes Atlas, 9th edition', *Diabetes Research and Clinical Practice*, November 2019, 157 (107843), https://doi.org/10.1016/j.diabres.2019.107843.
7. Bommer, Christian et al., 'The global economic burden of diabetes in adults aged 20–79 years: A cost-of-illness study', *The Lancet Diabetes & Endocrinology*, June 2017, 5(6), https://doi.org/10.1016/S2213-8587(17)30097-9.
8. Mui, Katie, 'The GoodRx List Price Index Reveals the Rising Cost of All Diabetes Treatments–Not Just Insulin', *GoodRx Health*, 10 April 2019, https://bit.ly/3vZ0R8L. Accessed on 27 October 2021.
9. Ramachandran, A. et al., 'Increasing Expenditure on Health Care Incurred by Diabetic Subjects in a Developing Country: A study from India', *Diabetes Care*, February 2007, 30(2): 252–56, https://doi.org/10.2337/dc06-0144.
10. Singla, R. et al., 'Drug Prescription Patterns and Cost Analysis of Diabetes Therapy in India: Audit of an Endocrine Practice', *Indian J Endocrinol Metab*, 2019; 23(1): 40–45, doi:10.4103/ijem.IJEM_646_18.
11. Ahlqvist, Emma et al., 'Novel subgroups of adult-onset diabetes and their association with outcomes: a data-driven cluster analysis of six variables', *The Lancet Diabetes & Endocronology*, May 2018, 6(5): P361–69, https://doi.org/10.1016/S2213-8587(18)30051-2.
12. Sussman, J.B. et al., 'Rates of Deintensification of Blood Pressure and Glycemic Medication Treatment Based on Levels of Control and Life Expectancy in Older Patients With Diabetes Mellitus', *JAMA Intern Med*, December 2015,175(12):1942–49, doi: 10.1001/jamainternmed.2015.5110.

13 Harrison, Leonard C. et al., 'Does rotavirus turn on type 1 diabetes?' *PLOS Pathogens*, 15(10): e1007965, DOI: 10.1371/journal.ppat.1007965.
14 Cole, David K. et al., 'Hotspot autoimmune T cell receptor binding underlies pathogen and insulin peptide cross-reactivity', *Journal of Clinical Investigation*, 2016, DOI: 10.1172/JCI85679.
15 Pellegrini, S. et al., 'Duodenal Mucosa of Patients with Type 1 Diabetes Shows Distinctive Inflammatory Profile and Microbiota', *The Journal of Clinical Endocrinology & Metabolism*, May 2017, 102(5): 1468–77, https://doi.org/10.1210/jc.2016-3222.
16 In ketoacidosis, the body breaks down fats for fuel, generating a dangerous build-up of toxic ketone acids, which can lead to diabetic coma and death.
17 International Diabetes Federation (IDF) Diabetes Atlas, 8th Edition (2017), www.diabetesatlas.org.
18 Hypo or hypoglycaemia occurs when blood sugar levels become abnormally low and is a potentially serious condition. Hypoglycemia can strike people with diabetes, type 1 or type 2, if they don't eat enough or if they take too much insulin.
19 Dr Ashok Seth is the chairman of Fortis Escorts Heart Institute, New Delhi, the chairman of Fortis Healthcare Medical Council, an adjunct professor of Cardiology at J.N. Medical College (Aligarh Muslim University) and is on the National Board of Examinations.
20 King, Dana E., 'C-Reactive Protein and Glycemic Control in Adults with Diabetes', *Diabetes Care*, May 2003, 26(5): 1535–39, https://doi.org/10.2337/diacare.26.5.1535.
21 McFadden, Johnjoe, 'The power in Rooney's foot', *The Guardian*, 6 June 2006, https://bit.ly/3nvr0rY. Accessed on 28 October 2021.
22 Neruda, Pablo, *Ode to the Liver*, 1956; Arrese, M., 'The liver in poetry: Neruda's "Ode to the liver",' *Liver International*, August 2008, 28(7): 901–05.
23 Pearson-Stuttard, J. et al., 'Trends in predominant causes of death in individuals with and without diabetes in England from 2001 to 2018: an epidemiological analysis of linked primary care records', *The Lancet: Diabetes and Endocrinology*, March 2021, 9(3): P165–173, DOI: https://doi.org/10.1016/S2213-8587(20)30431-9.
24 Kim, Jung-whan and Chi V. Dang, 'Cancer's Molecular Sweet Tooth and the Warburg Effect', *Cancer Research*, September 2006, 66(18), https://doi.org/10.1158/0008-5472.CAN-06-1501.

25. Thompson, Craig, 'Fueling Cancer', *Cell Press*, September 2015, 1(1): P12–13, https://doi.org/10.1016/j.trecan.2015.08.005.
26. Garber, Ken, 'Energy Boost: The Warburg Effect Returns in a New Theory of Cancer', *JNCI: Journal of the National Cancer Institute*, 15 December 2004, 96(24): 1805–06, https://doi.org/10.1093/jnci/96.24.1805.

Chapter 6: Sugar and the Slow Burn

1. Mohanty, P. et al., 'Glucose Challenge Stimulates Reactive Oxygen Species (ROS) Generation by Leucocytes', *The Journal of Clinical Endocrinology & Metabolism*, August 2008, 5(8): 2970–73, https://doi.org/10.1210/jcem.85.8.6854.
2. Shaw, Jonathan, 'Raw and Red-Hot: Could inflammation be the cause of myriad chronic conditions?' *Harvard Magazine*, May–June 2019, https://bit.ly/38Ig5Yj. Accessed on 11 April 2022.
3. Burhans, M.S. et al., 'Contribution of adipose tissue inflammation to the development of type 2 diabetes mellitus', *Compr Physiol*, June 2019, 9(1): 1–58, doi:10.1002/cphy.c170040.
4. Lafontan M., 'Fat cells: Afferent and efferent messages define new approaches to treat obesity', *Annu Rev Pharmacol Toxicol*, 2005, 45: 119–46, doi: 10.1146/annurev.pharmtox.45.120403.095843. PMID: 15822173.
5. Pollan, Michael, 'Unhappy Meals', *The New York Times*, 28 January 2007, https://nyti.ms/3pLBOFg. Accessed on 28 October 2021.
6. World Health Organization, *Globalization, Diets and Noncommunicable Diseases*, World Health Organization, 2003, https://apps.who.int/iris/handle/10665/42609. Accessed 11 April 2022.
7. Anette, Christ et al., 'Western diet and the Immune System: An Inflammatory Connection', *Immunity*, 19 November 2019, 51(5): P794–811, https://doi.org/10.1016/j.immuni.2019.09.020.
8. Cordain, Loren et al., 'Origins and evolution of the Western diet: Health implications for the 21st century', *Am J Clin Nutr*, 2005, 81: 341–54, https://academic.oup.com/ajcn/article/81/2/341/4607411.
9. Newens, K.J. and J. Walton, 'A review of sugar consumption from nationally representative dietary surveys across the world',

Journal of Human Nutrition and Dietetics, April 2016, 29(2): 225–40, https://doi.org/110.1111/jhn.12338.

10. Furman, David et al., 'Chronic inflammation in the etiology of disease across the life span', *Nature Medicine*, December 2019, 25:1822–1832, doi.org/10.1038/s41591-019-0675-0.

11. Seshadri, K.G., 'Obesity: A Venusian story of Paleolithic proportions', *Indian J Endocrinol Metab.*, January–February 2012, 16(1): 134–35, doi: 10.4103/2230-8210.91208.

12. Landrigan, P.J., et al., 'The *Lancet* Commission on pollution and health', *The Lancet*, October 2017, 391(10119), DOI: https://doi.org/10.1016/S0140-6736(17)32345-0.

13. Rajagopalan, Sanjay et al., 'Metabolic effects of air pollution exposure and reversibility', *Journal of Clinical Investigation*, 2 November 2020, 130(11): 6034–40, https://doi.org/10.1172/JCI137315.

14. 'The 2016 global and national burden of diabetes mellitus attributable to PM2·5 air pollution', *The Lancet Planetary Health*, July 2018, 2(7): E301–E312, https://doi.org/10.1016/S2542-5196(18)30140-2.

15. Puett, R.C. et al., 'Are Particulate Matter Exposures Associated with Risk of Type 2 Diabetes?' *Environmental Health Perspectives*, March 2011, 119(3): 384–89, https://doi.org/10.1289/ehp.1002344.

16. Tarantino, G. et al., 'Exposure to ambient air particulate matter and non-alcoholic fatty liver disease', *World J Gastroenterol*, July 2013, 19(25): 3951–56, doi: 10.3748/wjg.v19.i25.3951.

17. Yin, P. et al., 'The effect of air pollution on deaths, disease burden, and life expectancy across China and its provinces, 1990–2017: An analysis for the Global Burden of Disease Study 2017', *The Lancet Planetary Health*, 1 September 2020, 4(9): E386–E398, https://doi.org/10.1016/S2542-5196(20)30161-3.

18. PM 1, PM 2.5, PM 10, SO2, NO2 and O3 are ambient air pollutants. PM stands for particulate matter of aerodynamic diameter less than 1 μm (micrometre), 2.5 μm and 10 μm, respectively. Ozone (O3), nitrogen dioxide (NO2), sulfur dioxide (SO2) and carbon monoxide (CO) are the other major environmental factors causing disease and death worldwide.

19. Tan, Hwei-Ee et al., 'The Gut–Brain Axis Mediates Sugar Preference', *Nature*, 15 April 2020, 580: 511–16,

https://doi.org/10.1038/s41586-020-2199-7; Fernandes, Ana B. et al., 'Postingestive Modulation of Food Seeking Depends on Vagus-Mediated Dopamine Neuron Activity', 3 June 2020, *Neuron*, 106(5), https://doi.org/10.1016/j.neuron.2020.03.009.
20. Dias, Jenny Pena et al., 'The longitudinal association of changes in diurnal cortisol features with fasting glucose: MESA', *Psychoneuroendocrinology*, 2020, 119: 104698, ISSN 0306–4530, https://doi.org/10.1016/j.psyneuen.2020.104698.
21. Jaret, Peter, 'The Surprising Benefits of Stress', *Greater Good Magazine*, 20 October 2015, https://bit.ly/3EluANs. Accessed on 18 April 2022.
22. Pavlov, V.A. et al., 'The vagus nerve and the inflammatory reflex—linking immunity and metabolism', *Nature Reviews Endocrinology*, December 2012, 8(12): 743–54, https://doi.org/10.1038/nrendo.2012.189.
23. Franceschi, C. et al., 'Inflammaging: A new immune–metabolic viewpoint for age-related diseases', *Nature Reviews Endocrinology*, July 2018, 14: 576–90, https://doi.org/10.1038/s41574-018-0059-4.
24. The Nobel Prize in Physiology or Medicine 2009 was presented jointly to Elizabeth H. Blackburn, Carol W. Greider and Jack W. Szostak for their discovery on the way chromosomes are protected by telomeres and the enzyme telomerase. For more information, see 'Illustrated Presentation', The Nobel Prize, https://bit.ly/3bljhqW. Accessed on 28 October 2021.
25. Twohig-Bennett, C. and A. Jones, 'The health benefits of the great outdoors: A systematic review and meta-analysis of greenspace exposure and health outcomes', *Environmental Research*, October 2018, 166: 628–37, https://doi.org/10.1016/j.envres.2018.06.030.
26. Kalyani, B.G. et al., 'Neurohemodynamic correlates of "OM" chanting: A pilot functional magnetic resonance imaging study', *International Journal of Yoga*, January–June 2011, 4(1): 3–6, https://doi.org/10.4103/0973-6131.78171.

Chapter 7: The Great Nutrition Transition

1. Dr Ambrish Mithal is the chairman and head of Endocrinology and Diabetes at Max Healthcare, Saket, New Delhi.
2. Datta, Damayanti, 'Anna is in a stable condition but his

parameters are all downhill', *India Today,* 26 August 2011.
3   Nair, Aditya, '11-year-old Girl Dies in Jharkhand after being Denied Ration over Aadhaar Linking', News18, 17 October 2017, https://bit.ly/3jJcDiv. Accessed on 29 October 2021.
4   Grebmer, Klaus von et al., 'Global Hunger Index: The Challenge of Hidden Hunger', International Food Policy Research Institute, Welthungerhilfe and Concern Worldwide, October 2014, Chapter 3.
5   Sánchez-Moreno, C. et al., 'Stroke: roles of B vitamins, homocysteine and antioxidants', *Nutrition Research Reviews,* June 2009, 22(1): 49–67, https://doi.org/10.1017/S0954422409990023.
6   Rao, R.H., 'The role of undernutrition in the pathogenesis of diabetes mellitus', *Diabetes Care,* 1984, 7: 595–601.
7   'The 2021 Global Nutrition Report: The state of global nutrition', Development Initiatives, Bristol, UK, https://globalnutritionreport.org/reports/2021-global-nutrition-report. Accessed on 11 April 2022.
8   '2021 Global Hunger Index: Hunger and food systems in conflict settings', Bonn/Dublin, Concern Worldwide and Welthungerhilfe, October 2021.
9   Ramachandran, A. et al., 'Temporal changes in prevalence of diabetes and impaired glucose tolerance associated with lifestyle transition occurring in the rural population in India', *Diabetologia,* May 2004, 47: 860–65.
10 Dr Viswanathan Mohan, president and chief of Diabetes Research, Madras Diabetes Research Foundation, as well as chairman and chief diabetologist, Dr. Mohan's Diabetes Specialities Centre, Chennai, India.
11 Kumar, S. et al., 'Perceptions about Varieties of Brown Rice: A Qualitative Study from Southern India', *Journal of the American Dietetic Association,* October 2011, 111(10): 1517–22, https://doi.org/10.1016/j.jada.2011.07.002.
12 Balaji, Bhavadharini et al., 'White Rice Intake and Incident Diabetes: A Study of 132,373 Participants in 21 Countries', *Diabetes Care,* November 2020, 43(11): 2643–50, https://doi.org/10.2337/dc19-2335.
13 Micha, Renata et al., 'Global Nutrition Report: Action on Equity to

End Malnutrition. Technical Report', Nina Behrman (ed) (2020) Development Initiatives, Bristol, [Monograph].
14. Baker, P. and S. Friel, 'Processed Foods and the Nutrition Transition: Evidence from Asia', *Obesity Reviews*, July 2014, 15(7): 564–77, https://doi.org/10.1111/obr.12174.
15. Kesavan, P.C. and M.S. Swaminathan, 'Modern Technologies for Sustainable Food and Nutrition Security', *Current Science*, 25 November 2018, 115(10): 1876–83.
16. Das, Raju J., 'Geographical Unevenness of India's Green Revolution', *Journal of Contemporary Asia*, 1999, 29(2): 167–86, https://doi.org/10.1080/00472339980000301.
17. Vidal, John, 'Norman Borlaug: Humanitarian hero or menace to society?' *The Guardian*, 1 April 2014, https://bit.ly/31cPE9n. Accessed on 29 October 2021.
18. *Diet Nutrition and the Prevention of Chronic Diseases*, Report of a Joint WHO/FAO Expert Consultation, World Health Organization, Geneva, 2003, p. 16.

Chapter 8: A Virus That Loves Sugar

1. Angiotensin-Converting Enzyme 2 (ACE2) receptors are found in the lungs, the cardiovascular system, kidneys and the brain.
2. Logette, E. et al., 'A Machine-Generated View of the Role of Blood Glucose Levels in the Severity of COVID-19', *Frontiers in Public Health*, 28 July 2021, doi.org/10.3389/fpubh.2021.695139.
3. Deng M. et al., 'Can We Reduce Mortality of COVID-19 if we do Better in Glucose Control?' *Medicine in Drug Discovery*, September 2020, 7(100048), https://doi.org/10.1016/j.medidd.2020.100048.
4. Scudellari, Megan, 'How the coronavirus infects cells—and why Delta is so dangerous', *Nature*, 28 July 2021, 595: 640–44, https://doi.org/10.1038/d41586-021-02039-y.
5. Codo, A.C. et al., 'Elevated Glucose Levels Favor SARS-CoV-2 Infection and Monocyte Response through a HIF-1a/Glycolysis-Dependent Axis', *Cell Metabolism*, September 2020, 32(3): 437–46, https://doi.org/10.1016/j.cmet.2020.07.007.
6. Zhou, B. et al., 'Worldwide trends in hypertension prevalence and progress in treatment and control from 1990 to 2019: a

pooled analysis of 1201 population-representative studies with 104 million participants', *The Lancet*, NCD Risk Factor Collaboration (NCD-RisC), 11 September 2021, 398 (10304): 957–80, DOI: https://doi.org/10.1016/S0140-6736(21)01330-1; International Diabetes Foundation (IDF) Diabetes Atlas; Abdul-Aziz, A. Ahmad et al., 'Tackling the Burden of Cardiovascular Diseases in India', *Circulation: Cardiovascular Quality and Outcomes*, March 2019, 12(4), https://doi.org/10.1161/CIRCOUTCOMES.118.005195.

7 Zhang, J. et al., 'Impaired Fasting Glucose and Diabetes are Related to Higher Risks of Complications and Mortality among Patients with Coronavirus Disease 2019', *Front Endocrinol*, July 2020, 11:525, doi: 10.3389/fendo.2020.00525.

8 Ceriello, A., 'Hyperglycemia and the worse prognosis of COVID-19. Why a fast blood glucose control should be mandatory', *Diabetes Res Clin Pract*, May 2020, 163:108186, doi: 10.1016/j.diabres.2020.108186.

9 Wargny, M. et al., 'Predictors of hospital discharge and mortality in patients with diabetes and COVID-19: updated results from the nationwide CORONADO study', *Diabetologia*, February 2021, 64: 778–94, https://doi.org/10.1007/s00125-020-05351-w.

10 Singh, A.K. and A. Misra, 'Impact of COVID-19 and Comorbidities on Health and Economics: Focus on Developing Countries and India', *Diabetes & Metabolic Syndrome: Clinical Research & Reviews*, November–December 2020, 14(6): 1625–30, https://doi.org/10.1016/j.dsx.2020.08.032.

11 Heianza, Y. et al., 'Fasting glucose and HbA1c levels as risk factors for the development of hypertension in Japanese individuals: Toranomon hospital health management center study 16 (TOPICS 16)', *Journal of Human Hypertension*, 29 (2015): 254–59, https://doi.org/10.1038/jhh.2014.77.

12 García-Puig, J. et al., 'Glucose Metabolism in Patients with Essential Hypertension', *The American Journal of Medicine*, April 2006, 119(4): 318–26, https://doi.org/10.1016/j.amjmed.2005.09.010.

13 Carnevale Schianca, G.P. et al., 'Impaired glucose metabolism in hypertensive patients with/without the metabolic syndrome', *European Journal of International Medicine*, May 2014, 25(5): 477–81, https://doi.org/10.1016/j.ejim.2014.04.006.

14 'CDC updates, expands list of people at risk of severe COVID-19

illness', CDC Press Release, 25 June 2020.
15. For more information, please visit: http://covidiab.e-dendrite.com/.
16. Ghosh, Amerta et al., 'Glycemic parameters in patients with new-onset diabetes during COVID-19 pandemic are more severe than in patients with new-onset diabetes before the pandemic: NOD COVID India Study', *Diabetes & Metabolic Syndrome: Clinical Research & Reviews,* January–February 2021, 15(1): 215–20, https://doi.org/10.1016/j.dsx.2020.12.033.
17. Ghosh, Amerta, 'Effects of nationwide lockdown during COVID-19 epidemic on lifestyle and other medical issues of patients with type 2 diabetes in north India', *Diabetes & Metabolic Syndrome: Clinical Research & Reviews,* September 2020, 14(5): 917–20, https://doi.org/10.1016/j.dsx.2020.05.044.
18. Arora, Umang et al., 'Novel risk factors for Coronavirus disease-associated mucormycosis (CAM): a case control study during the outbreak in India', *MedRxiv* preprint, July 2021, https://doi.org/10.1101/2021.07.24.21261040.
19. Dhar, D. and A. Mohanty, 'Gut microbiota and Covid-19— possible link and implications', *Virus Res.* 2020 August; 285:198018. doi: 10.1016/j.virusres.2020.198018.
20. Holshue, Michelle L. et al., 'First Case of 2019 Novel Coronavirus in the United States', *The New England Journal of Medicine,* March 2020, 382: 929–36; DOI: https://doi.org/10.1056/NEJMoa2001191.
21. Yeoh, Y.K. et al., 'Gut microbiota composition reflects disease severity and dysfunctional immune responses in patients with COVID-19', *Gut,* April 2021, 70: 698–706.
22. Chopra, Deepak and Rudolph E. Tanzi, 'The Planetary Biome: A New Theory of Life and Survival', *Deepak Chopra,* 6 September 2020, https://bit.ly/3CAObY3. Accessed on 1 November 2021.

Chapter 9: Eating with the Gods

1. Stevens, John, 'What kind of food did Sakyamuni Buddha eat?' *Journal of Indian and Buddhist Studies,* December 1985, 34 (1), http://buddhism.lib.ntu.edu.tw/DLMBS/en/journal/journaldetail.jsp?seq=1831&comefrom=bookdetail.
2. Joshi, C.V., 'Life and Teachings', in *2500 Years of Buddhism,*

P.V. Bapat (ed.), Publications Division, Ministry of Information and Broadcasting, Government of India, 1959, Chapter III.
3   Warren, Henry Clarke, *Buddhism in Translations*, Harvard University Press, Cambridge, 1896, pp. 71–74.
4   Strode, Muriel, 'The Buddha's Hymn of Victory', *The Open Court Journal*, Vol. 1 (1905), Issue No. 1: 5–39.
5   Tu, Thich Nhat (ed.), *Family and Society: A Buddhist Perspective*, Hong Duc Publishing House, Hanoi, 2019, p. 198.
6   Willett, W. et al., 'Food in the Anthropocene: the EAT–*Lancet* Commission on healthy diets from sustainable food systems', *Lancet*, 393(10170) (published online 16 January): 447–92, https://doi.org/10.1016/S0140-6736(18)31788-4.
7   Horner, I.B (trans.), *The Book of the Discipline, Vinaya-Pitaka*, Vol. IV, Mahāvagga, The Pali Text Society, Lancaster, 1951, p. 105, p. 166.
8   de Cabo, Rafael and Mark P. Mattson, 'Effects of Intermittent Fasting on Health, Aging, and Disease', *New England Journal of Medicine*, December 2019, doi/full/10.1056/NEJMx190038.
9   Prakash, Om, *Food and Drink in Ancient India: From Earliest Times to c. 1200 A.D*, Munshi Manohar Lal, Delhi, 1961, pp. 7–33.
10 Nishimura Naoko, 'Amiksa and Payasya: Processing of fermented milk in ancient India', *Journal of Indian and Buddhist Studies*, March 2011, 59(3).
11 Fung Teresa T., et al., 'Whole-grain intake and the risk of type 2 diabetes: A prospective study in men', *The American Journal of Clinical Nutrition*, September 2002, 76(3): 535–40.
12 Wastyk, Hannah C. et al., 'Gut-microbiota-targeted diets modulate human immune status', *Cell*, August 2021: 184(16): 4137–53, https://doi.org/10.1016/j.cell.2021.06.019.
13 Warraich, Haider, 'Evolution Gave Us Heart Disease. We're Not Stuck with it', *The New York Times*, 6 August 2019, https://nyti.ms/3GGQWcU. Accessed on 2 November 2021.
14 'Baiga Tribe of Madhya Pradesh', *The Reflective Indian*, 9 January 2013, https://bit.ly/3KR0bca. Accessed on 19 April 2022.
15 'English rendering of PM's speech at the presentation of Yoga Awards', Press Information Bureau, Government of India, Prime Minister's Office, 30 August 2019, https://bit.ly/3mUSbNU. Accessed on 2 November 2021.

16. Kumar, D. et al., 'Scope of Food: Barley Research and Development in India', *Wheat and Barley Research* (2018), 10(3): 166–72, doi.org/10.25174/2249-4065/2018/84878.
17. Mondal, Debayan et al., 'Evaluation of indigenous aromatic rice cultivars from sub-Himalayan Terai region of India for nutritional attributes and blast resistance', *Scientific Reports*, 2021, 11 (4786).
18. Ahuja, Uma et al., 'Rice: A Nutraceutical', *Asian Agri-History*, 2008, 12(2): 93–108.
19. Wastyk, Hannah C. et al., 'Gut-microbiota-targeted diets modulate human immune status', *Cell*, 2021, 184(16): 4137–53, https://doi.org/10.1016/j.cell.2021.06.019.
20. In July 2021, Kishwar Chowdhury, a contestant on Masterchef Australia, presented an elaborate version of panta bhaat, which she called 'Smoked Rice Water'.
21. Goswami, Gunajit et al., 'Fermentation Reduces Anti-Nutritional Content and Increases Mineral Availability in *Poita bhat*', *Asian Journal of Chemistry*, 2016, 28(9): 1929–32, https://doi.org/10.14233/ajchem.2016.19820.
22. Pradhan, Hemata, 'Pakhala boosts immunity, finds city AIIMS study', *The Times of India*, 8 July 2021.

Made in the USA
Monee, IL
03 May 2026